THE IRRITABLE BOWEL STRESS BOOK

ROSEMARY NICOL lives in Somerset, and is married with four chi Like a Dream – the Know Abou Coping Successfully rritable Bowel Diet

Overcoming Common Problems Series

For a full list of titles please contact
Sheldon Press, Marylebone Road, London NW1 4DU

Beating Job Burnout
DR DONALD SCOTT

Beating the Blues
SUSAN TANNER AND JILLIAN
BALL

Being the Boss
STEPHEN FITZSIMON

Birth Over Thirty
SHEILA KITZINGER

Body Language
How to read others' thoughts by their
gestures
ALLAN PEASE

Bodypower
DR VERNON COLEMAN

Bodysense
DR VERNON COLEMAN

Calm Down
How to cope with frustration and anger
DR PAUL HAUCK

Changing Course
How to take charge of your career
SUE DYSON AND STEPHEN HOARE

Comfort for Depression
JANET HORWOOD

Complete Public Speaker
GYLES BRANDRETH

**Coping Successfully with Your Child's
Asthma**
DR PAUL CARSON

**Coping Successfully with Your Hyperactive
Child**
DR PAUL CARSON

**Coping Successfully with Your Irritable
Bowel**
ROSEMARY NICOL

Coping with Anxiety and Depression
SHIRLEY TRICKETT

Coping with Blushing
DR ROBERT EDELMANN

Coping with Cot Death
SARAH MURPHY

Coping with Depression and Elation
DR PATRICK McKEON

Coping with Stress
DR GEORGIA WITKIN-LANOIL

Coping with Suicide
DR DONALD SCOTT

Coping with Thrush
CAROLINE CLAYTON

Curing Arthritis – The Drug-Free Way
MARGARET HILLS

Curing Arthritis Diet Book
MARGARET HILLS

**Curing Coughs, Colds and Flu – The
Drug-Free Way**
MARGARET HILLS

Curing Illness – The Drug-Free Way
MARGARET HILLS

Depression
DR PAUL HAUCK

Divorce and Separation
ANGELA WILLANS

Don't Blame Me!
How to stop blaming yourself
and other people
TONY GOUGH

The Epilepsy Handbook
SHELAGH McGOVERN

**Everything You Need to Know about
Adoption**
MAGGIE JONES

**Everything You Need to Know about
Contact Lenses**
DR ROBERT YOUNGSON

**Everything You Need to Know about
Osteoporosis**
ROSEMARY NICOL

Overcoming Common Problems Series

Overcoming Common Problems Series

Overcoming Common Problems

THE IRRITABLE BOWEL STRESS BOOK

Rosemary Nicol

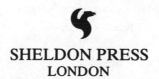

SHELDON PRESS
LONDON

First published in Great Britain in 1991
Sheldon Press, SPCK, Marylebone Road, London NW1 4DU

© Rosemary Nicol 1991

616.34

British Library Cataloguing in Publication Data

Nicol, Rosemary
    The irritable bowel stress book.
    I. Title
    616.34

ISBN 0–85969–637–5

Photoset by Deltatype Ltd, Ellesmere Port, Cheshire
Printed in Great Britain by Courier International Ltd, East Kilbride

Contents

Acknowledgements

The extracts from the Workers' Educational Association pack on Women and Health are reproduced by permission of the Health Education Authority. The Holmes–Rahe Life Stress Inventory is reproduced by permission of Pergamon Press.

Illustrations: p. 58 'Salute to the Sun' is reproduced from *Yoga* by Sophy Hoare by permission of Macdonald & Co; p. 61 Justin Salinger; pp. 40, 45, 56 John Erasmus; p. 43 Alasdair Smith.

1

Irritable Bowel Syndrome: What is it?

'The irritable bowel syndrome remains a clinical conundrum. It is a syndrome that lacks a clear definition. . . . There are no known clinical tests that will confirm or refute the diagnosis with certainty, and there is no specific therapy for the condition. Many attempts have been made to establish both the reality and the unity of the syndrome; all have, to a greater or lesser extent, failed.' from *Digestion*, *45*, 1990

The language from this journal may be full of medical terminology, but the message is clear: irritable bowel syndrome (IBS) is an enigma, a puzzle. No one yet knows for sure what it is, how to test for it, or how to treat it successfully.

This is a pity, because about one-third of the general population have the symptoms at some time or another, and about 13% have them regularly. It accounts for half of all patients seen by gastroenterologists, and is a condition that can cause pain, embarrassment, a loss of self-confidence and self-esteem, and for many people may lead to days off work, a limited diet and a restricted social life.

The exact cause of irritable bowel syndrome is not yet known, but most people can trace theirs back to one of the following:

- an attack of gastro-enteritis – 'holiday tummy' – which may make the intestines over-reactive and sensitive;
- a long course of antibiotics, which may alter the delicate balance of natural beneficial bacteria in the body;
- an abdominal or pelvic operation;
- a stressful time, such as divorce, threat of redundancy, unemployment, exams, or problems in a personal relationship.

It is this last aspect of irritable bowel syndrome that this book is about.

In his Foreword to my earlier book, *Coping Successfully with Your Irritable Bowel* (Sheldon 1988), Mr Andrew Gough, a consultant gastroenterologist, says, 'To regard IBS as just a disorder of the bowel is just not tenable these days. It is surely an expression of personality, stress and environment.'

If you can develop techniques to manage the stressful parts of your life you will have a much better chance of coping successfully with your irritable bowel syndrome; the rest of this book will give you lots of ideas for doing that.

So what exactly is irritable bowel syndrome?

When used as a medical term, *irritable* doesn't mean that you are bad-tempered, irascible and difficult to live with! It just means that some part of you (in this case your bowel) is over-reacting to something. That something could be a particular food, or an antibiotic, or the overfulness of constipation, or something in your life that is sending messages that make it behave abnormally.

The *bowel* is the intestines, also known as the gut, and includes both the small and the large intestines – about 40 feet (12 metres) of colon, rectum, and other lengths of tubing, whose job is to propel food from the stomach to the rectum, extracting all the goodness out of it on the way, and storing the final waste products until it can be passed out of the body through the anus (back passage). It is your bowel that is over-reacting, and propelling the food in an irregular way.

A *syndrome* is a collection of symptoms all together, and IBS certainly has plenty of those. The symptoms that nowadays are recognized as typical of the condition are:

- abdominal pain (i.e. pain in the tummy), usually low down on the left, or possibly centre or right;
- constipation, usually with stomach pain, and small lumpy stools like 'rabbit droppings';
- alternating diarrhoea and constipation, often in an unpredictable and erratic fashion;
- an abdomen that looks or feels bloated and distended;

- feeling 'full of wind';
- passing mucus with the stools, or by itself;
- in addition, it generally becomes worse during periods of stress, and may disappear completely at other times.

Not content with all this, you may also have an even longer list of other symptoms:

Digestive
heartburn
nausea
feeling full early in a meal
an unpleasant taste in the mouth
loss of appetite
regurgitating acid
belching
difficulty in swallowing
rumblings and gurglings
occasional vomiting

Bowel and bladder
passing urine often
needing to go to the toilet urgently
after a bowel movement feeling there is more to come

States of mind
tiredness or lethargy
anxiety
irritation
loss of concentration
mild depression and weeping
lack of 'sparkle'

Physical
back pain
sleeping difficulties
feeling hot behind the eyes (like 'flu)

headache, possibly with sweating, flushes and faintness
reduced sex drive

Extra problems for women
painful intercourse
painful periods
feeling the symptoms get worse around the time of a period

But don't despair, there is still a great deal you can do to help yourself. Whatever the main symptoms of your IBS, there is a great weight of evidence to show that *a reduction in the symptoms is more likely in those who are able to acknowledge the role of stress in their IBS and take steps to reduce it than in those who are not.*

For a great many people, learning how to cope with the stress side of life is more effective in treating IBS than the bulk laxatives, anti-spasmodic drugs and advice on a high-fibre diet that are the doctor's first line of attack. The doctor's methods will work for many people, but unfortunately IBS is a chronic condition that is treated with lots of different drugs without a particularly good success rate. At least stress management is something you can do for yourself, and by doing it you will begin to feel that you are controlling your insides rather than the other way round.

2

Are You Under Stress?

In *Coping Successfully with Your Irritable Bowel*, you may remember a prehistoric character called *Homo Sapiens*. He lived in a cave, and from time to time he came across the greater four-toed mammoth. On a good day, he would see the mammoth and think, 'This will keep me and the missus in meat and fur for many a moon. I will chase after it.' On a bad day he would see the mammoth walking purposefully towards him with a glint in its eye that said, 'Ah, lunch'. Either way, he would need to run.

Whether *Homo Sapiens* runs towards or away from the mammoth, his body will gear itself for a decidedly stressful few minutes. His brain sends messages to his adrenal glands to produce lots of adrenalin; this causes vital changes to take place to give him a better chance of survival. The blood will drain from his skin and digestive organs, to give more resources to his muscles. Sugars and fats will be released into his blood to provide much needed energy for all that running. He will breathe faster, so more oxygen is made available to burn up the sugar and fat and make it useful quickly. His pupils will enlarge to give him better vision. His blood will thicken so it will coagulate quickly if he is wounded. And his blood pressure will rise as his heart pumps away like crazy keeping his whole body working in overdrive.

Mr *Homo Sapiens* probably saw it as a matter of life or death. Modern physiologists call it the fight-or-flight response, but it's all the same thing – a response to a stressful situation – only nowadays there's less fight or flight, and more just sitting around feeling angry or bored or frustrated. We still get the same responses – the extra adrenalin, the release of fats or sugars, the thickened blood, the close-down of the digestive system, the raised blood pressure – but no physical activity to put it to good use. So the blood remains thicker for some time, fats and sugars hang around in the bloodstream, the heart takes time to return to its normal pressure – the perfect scenario for coronary heart disease and other stress-related illnesses.

The first thing is to recognize how stress affects you. It's not usually too difficult to see that your spouse, your boss, or your friend is stressed. Equally they can probably see what state you are in. But can you?

'Under stress? Me? Good gracious, no, of course I'm not. Whatever makes you think that? Michael is, that's for sure – you can tell by the amount he smokes; and Bill had that heart attack last month so I expect he is; and Janet's biting her nails again. But me? – certainly not, I'm coping just fine.'

Why is it, you may ask yourself, that it's all right for other people to be showing signs of stress, but not for you? Many people are unwilling to admit to being stressed in case others see them as weak, ineffectual, or unable to cope. They feel that they should be seen as strong and capable, a tower of strength to others, someone to lean on who can put up with whatever life throws at them and survive unscathed. I hope that by the end of this book you will feel it's all right to be vulnerable, to give in sometimes, and to have a condition that may be triggered by stress.

Imagine you are quietly living your life when suddenly you get blinding headaches, or disturbed vision, or severe chest pains. You would take it seriously, go straight to the doctor, submit to tests, take any drugs you are given, and probably make some changes in your way of life to make sure it didn't happen again. But instead, the chances are that your IBS came on fairly gradually – a bit of indigestion, minor abdominal pains, mild 'food poisoning', nothing to bother about much. So you let it go on and on, not taking it seriously, not making any changes, because the symptoms were not much more than a nuisance.

However if your IBS is triggered by stress, then ignoring what your body is trying to tell you can make the condition worse, until it becomes really painful, unpleasant, embarrassing, and spoils your enjoyment of life. Symptoms are signs, the body's way of telling you something is wrong, and emotional symptoms are just as important as physical ones. If you develop severe abdominal pain and start vomiting, it could be appendicitis. If you try to cover up the body's warning signs with pain killers or indigestion tablets you could develop peritonitis, and in extreme cases that could be fatal. Ignoring emotional warning signs can be just as serious.

Although stress is not as dramatic as appendicitis, it too has its own signs by which the body is trying to tell you 'There's something wrong here – please do something about it.'

There's no reason to be apologetic or defensive about having a stress-related condition. About half of all people who visit their GP have some kind of stress-related illness, so you are not at all unusual. But irritable bowel syndrome doesn't exactly make life a laugh-a-minute, and you'd probably be very glad to be rid of it.

Some people find conventional treatment works well. But for the majority of IBS sufferers, and especially those who have already had it for a few years, their insides may continue to bother them for a long time, and so they need to try several different approaches. The first approach is obviously treatment from your doctor, which may work well for you, or it may not. At the same time, you may change to a high-fibre diet, or, if this makes things worse, to a low-fibre diet; if you suspect particular foods may be the culprits, then a short-term exclusion diet should identify them for you (for more on diet, see my previous book *The Irritable Bowel Diet Book* (Sheldon 1990)).

But if none of these brings the improvement you had hoped for, what then? This is the point at which you might have to look yourself squarely in the eyes and consider whether the whole thing might be stress-related.

What is stress?

Stress is normal. It is even desirable (in the right place, at the right time, and in the right quantity). It can add spice to life, that extra something that gives you a buzz and makes you feel stretched, challenged, and stimulated.

In its positive form stress helps sportsmen and women to win, musicians and actors to perform better, artists of all kinds to be more creative, businessmen and women to meet deadlines, and all of us to avoid or survive dangerous situations.

Positive stress is when we feel confident we can overcome a challenge, exhilarated and invigorated by physical activity, winning the football pools, getting the job we wanted, starting a new love affair. Positive emotions increase our ability to withstand stress – excitement, happiness, confidence, pleasure, laughter, joy, love.

Negative stress isn't necessarily having a heavy work load, or working long hours, or having lots of responsibility and demands made on you, or even having a boring or repetitive job. Negative stress for *you* is what makes *you* physically or mentally unwell, those things that *your own personality* and past experiences find it hard to cope with, those things that get you stewed up inside because of your own attitudes and beliefs.

In the same way that positive emotions increase our ability to withstand stress, so negative emotions reduce this resistance. Emotions such as worry, guilt, anger, hostility, fear, anxiety, boredom and frustration are fine in small quantities, but if we build up too much of them we can end up in trouble. When stress first appears we usually note it with some physical or mental signs (increased heartbeat, excitement, etc), then we respond to the challenge and cope with the extra demand; so far, so good. But if we have too much, or in too short a time, or it goes on for too long, we become overburdened; if, finally, we ignore the warning signs (e.g. illness) the final stage is exhaustion, collapse, breakdown.

Who gets stressed?

Stress, like IBS, can occur at any stage of life:

Adolescents feel conflicts between the different expectations of themselves, their parents, their teachers and their friends. They want freedom and protection at the same time. Exams, sexual development, relationships with the opposite sex, disagreements with friends, peer pressure, insecurity, boredom, spots, body image, world issues, the environment . . . all these make adolescence a vulnerable time.

Early adulthood may bring pressures from getting married, starting (or failing to start) a family, mortgage repayments, finding a stable fulfilling job, parents' attitudes.

From about 35 to 45 we may be climbing the 'greasy pole', working long hours, coping with teenage children, responsibility at work, anxiety about promotion, possibly divorce. These are usually the years of maximum financial stretch and the worry that goes with it.

The mid-life crisis is well known: 'it's now or never', fear of redundancy or long-term illness, parents dying or becoming more dependent, children leaving home and becoming more independent, job insecurity, the continuing need for status, and so on.

All this makes stress a very individual thing. What upsets one person hardly bothers another. Examples of small-scale daily negative stress are: being stuck in a traffic jam, having a serious disagreement with a friend or neighbour, your secretary or assistant being off sick, a computer breaking down, getting a parking ticket, finding your hotel room has been double-booked, and lots more of the same.

How do you feel or behave when one of these happens to you? Do you, like an imaginary person we'll call Ray, lose your temper, behave in a rude or aggressive way, use obscenities in every sentence, threaten dire consequences to anyone involved, or even use physical violence? Or are you more like Tim, who is able to remain calm and courteous, talks in a quiet unthreatening way, makes the most of how things are, however annoying, and gets on with life without brooding about it all?

Ray is your ideal candidate for something as frightening as a stroke or heart attack, but because he is quite unable to recognize what he finds stressful, and even less able to handle it, he probably suffers from some form of stress-related illness, including IBS.

There is also a third character, we'll call her Penny. She is stuck in the same traffic jam as Ray and Tim, her hotel room is also over-booked, her assistant has phoned in sick, and her computer has broken down. What does she do? She feels just as angry as Ray, and yet, unlike Tim, she is unable to take it all in her stride. Inwardly she is furious with everyone, but she has been brought up to believe it is unladylike, unBritish, impolite,

9

and a form of weakness to let anyone know how she feels. All her emotions are tightly bottled up inside her; she is frightened of expressing annoyance, or disapproval, or anger. Perhaps her father had a violent temper, and she has seen the consequences it had on her mother and the rest of the family; perhaps as a child she was reprimanded for showing her feelings; perhaps her mother put up with whatever life threw at her, and Penny feels she should be able to do the same. Whatever the reason, Penny feels stress just as much as Ray does, and because she suffers from stress (revealed or concealed) she, too, suffers from a stress-related disease.

Some events are inherently stressful – being made redundant, being involved in a court case, family death or serious illness. But many other events are stressful, consciously or unconsciously, because we make them so – receiving criticism, being overtaken by a woman driver, anticipating an important event, seeing your spouse talking to an attractive member of the opposite sex, being left to do all the washing up. Whether you find these sort of things stressful depends on four components:

1) your basic temperament;
2) the extent to which you are able to deal with what life throws at you;
3) the level of stress you are already under;
4) whether you are a Type A personality (see Chapter 9)

You can't do much about (1), but there is quite a bit you can do about the other three. Other things also affect whether a particular event makes you feel stressed: your family background, how you were brought up to handle emotions and to think about different situations, your beliefs and attitudes, and your state of health. In any given situation (from being given a load of work to do in a short time to having an argument with a neighbour), person A may find it stressful, person B finds it tolerable, and person C may even thrive on it. Your life, and your digestive system would probably be a lot calmer if you could become more like person B.

So what do *you* need to do, for your general mental and

physical health, and particularly for your irritable bowel? There are five important steps to take:

First, recognize the signs that show *you* are under stress.

Second, be aware of what causes stress in your life.

Third, identify what you find relaxing, and develop some techniques for winding down.

Fourth, try, if possible, to remove or at least reduce the number of stressful things in your life.

Finally, anticipate and prepare yourself for those things you just have to put up with.

Recognizing signs of stress in yourself

Stress can show itself in many ways, physically, emotionally, or in the way you behave; we all feel stress differently. Look through this list, and tick anything that you experience when you feel stressed or under pressure:

Physical symptoms of stress

Tension in your muscles, e.g. shoulders, neck,
  jaw, hands   . . . .
Unexplained pains in your back or neck   . . . .
A knot in your stomach   . . . .
Nausea (feeling sick)   . . . .
Breathing fast or erratically, or breathlessness   . . . .
Holding your breath, or overbreathing   . . . .
Headaches or migraine   . . . .
Indigestion, or IBS symptoms   . . . .
Diarrhoea or constipation   . . . .
General aches and pains   . . . .
Dry mouth   . . . .
Menstrual problems   . . . .
Unusual sweating   . . . .
Chest palpitations   . . . .
Feeling restless or jumpy   . . . .
Difficulty sleeping   . . . .

Emotional signs of stress

Feeling depressed . . . .
Unable to cope . . . .
Anxious or nervous . . . .
Unusually irritable or angry . . . .
Irrational fears or feelings of panic . . . .
Weeping . . . .
Low self-image . . . .
Lack of self-confidence . . . .
Feeling inadequate . . . .
Feelings of hostility or resentment . . . .
Aggressiveness . . . .
Overcritical of yourself and others . . . .
Feeling 'I've had enough' . . . .
Tiredness, apathy, lack of energy . . . .
Feeling sorry for yourself . . . .
Worrying more about minor things . . . .
Difficulty in making rational judgements . . . .
Being unable to concentrate . . . .
Difficulty in making simple decisions . . . .
Getting things out of proportion . . . .
Feeling you can't talk to anyone about it . . . .
Becoming oversensitive to criticism . . . .

Behavioural signs of stress

Eating more, or less . . . .
Sleeping more, or less . . . .
Drinking or smoking more . . . .
Being unusually fussy about food . . . .
Talking much more or less than usual . . . .
Working much harder . . . .
Working much less . . . .
Losing interest in sex . . . .
Nail-biting . . . .
Fiddling continually with your hair . . . .
Licking your lips frequently . . . .
Drumming your fingers/jiggling your knees/
   tapping your feet . . . .

Reckless driving	. . . .
Becoming more accident-prone	. . . .

Be honest with yourself. You may not like to admit that you lose interest in sex, or drive recklessly, or lack self-confidence, or get things out of proportion. But if this is how stress shows itself in you, it is best to acknowledge it, so you can recognize the signs in good time – you might even see it coming before your gut does, and so avoid an attack of IBS. So take a deep breath, and (unless you are reading someone else's copy of the book!) put a tick against all those things that are peculiarly yours. Only when you can face up to it and recognize it will you be able and willing to take steps to change things.

After reading the rest of the book, and learning a few new techniques, you could come back to this list a few weeks later and find that you have managed to avoid some of those signs of stress. For example, if you drive more impatiently when things get on top of you, and if you can recognize this, then next time you shout at another motorist or cut the lights you could catch yourself in time and say: 'Hold on a minute, I'm obviously feeling stressed, so I'd better do something about it – soon'. With any luck, in a month's time you'll look back on four weeks of peaceful driving (and maybe a peaceful digestive system), and know that it works.

Other signs of stress

As you probably know, stress affects more than just your irritable bowel. It can cause many other complaints and diseases (although most of these can also have other causes):

- high blood pressure
- heart disease
- heart attacks
- strokes
- some forms of cancer
- some back pain
- tension headaches and migraine
- some allergies and asthma

- lowered resistance
- duodenal and gastric ulcers
- sexual problems
- hay fever
- rheumatoid arthritis
- diseases of the immune system
- impotence and frigidity
- skin conditions, including eczema and acne
- fatigue and lethargy

We all have an immune system which protects us against foreign substances by producing antibodies which seek out and destroy cells that are infected or cancerous, but stress reduces the ability of the immune system to do this. During stress, the levels of one of the antibodies known as immunoglobulin A (IgA for short) decrease, and this decrease can lower a person's resistance to infection. This could explain why we sometimes get a cold or a sore throat or some other illness after a period of stress.

As well as medical conditions, stress can also contribute to a whole host of social problems:

- marriage breakdown
- violence
- arguments
- absenteeism
- alcoholism
- drug dependence
- mental illness
- severe depression
- reckless driving

Although stress does have its positive side, for most of us in our modern world it tends to do more harm than good, and it doesn't do irritable bowel syndrome any good at all. It's unrealistic to expect that life will be a bed of roses all the time, but try to confine stress to one area of your life at a time. If your job is giving you aggravation, try to keep things quiet at home and in your leisure activities; if you have problems at home, don't stir things up at work and with your friends; and if your leisure activities are not going well do all you can to make home and work happy. It isn't always easy to do this; if you are in the middle of a divorce or separation it needs all your will-power to continue to do your job well, to feel at ease with your work colleagues, and to want to continue your usual leisure-time activities. If you are under threat of redundancy, this will probably cause extra anxieties at home, and you may also prefer not to tell your friends and this may put extra strains on those relationships. But home, work and leisure time are the three main areas of our lives, and we will be healthier in mind and body if each of them can be rich and fulfilling.

3

Stress and Your Irritable Bowel

'IBS patients are given diagnoses that appear to be vague, therapy that appears to be ineffective, and a prognosis that seems to be uncertain; meanwhile they are left with symptoms that suggest the possibility of undetected gastrointestinal disease.' from *Digestion, 45,* 1990.

The symptoms of IBS can be worrying (abdominal pain, erratic bowel habits, a tummy that is bloated and distended, passing mucus with or without stools), and it isn't surprising that many people do worry that they have some serious disease like colitis, or even cancer. Having started to worry, their anxiety can make the bowel behave even more irritably, and a vicious circle is set up.

So if you are worried about the assorted collection of symptoms that make up this strange syndrome, then it would be a good idea to go to your doctor and get it properly diagnosed; if you don't, the anxiety itself could be making it worse. Rest assured that IBS is not life-threatening, and there is no known connection between it and any serious bowel disease. It may be painful, embarrassing, disruptive to your daily life, and a real nuisance, but it won't kill you.

For many people, though, what will make it worse is stress. This could be any of the stresses of everyday living, or the stress of IBS itself. As you will know, having IBS can impose a whole range of extra stresses, particularly when you are away from home –

- Will there be a toilet where I'm going?
- How will I manage if there isn't one?
- What will other people think if I have to go to the toilet several times?

16

- Will the meal contain any of the things that disagree with me?
- Will my tummy rumbling, or passing wind, cause embarrassment?

It's quite possible to start worrying about any one of these things the moment you know you are going on holiday, or staying with friends, or having a business lunch or meeting in a strange place. You worry that you might feel tense, and then you start feeling tense. At that point the muscles in your large bowel start to contract extra-vigorously, you get abdominal pain, and possibly diarrhoea, and this just reinforces the original anxiety. It becomes all too easy to think, 'I can't do this, because if I do I'll get terrible pain and diarrhoea', although at this stage the pain and diarrhoea are being caused by nothing more than your worry about getting pain and diarrhoea. It is an interesting fact that many people start to get the symptoms of IBS *before* going out for a meal, suggesting that it is the anxiety about eating out rather than the food itself that is the root of the problem.

The majority of people with IBS don't see their doctor about it, and even manage to live fairly comfortably with the condition, but IBS patients who see their doctors regularly tend to have above-average levels of stress and anxiety, more general worries about their health, and find their IBS more disruptive to their lives than those who see their doctors seldom or not at all. It is easy for doctors to dismiss these patients as neurotic or obsessive or depressive, but this connection between regular visits to the doctor and a higher level of anxiety could be because their IBS really is more painful and more disruptive than that of someone who doesn't need to see the doctor so often. The medical article that the quotation at the beginning of this chapter is taken from says that these feelings of anxiety are '. . . consistent with the state of mind of a patient who is still searching for some rational explanation – and some effective therapy – for his or her symptoms' and it goes on to suggest that this is consistent with the suggestion that these worries are not the *cause* of IBS, but are the *result* of the IBS being ineffectively managed in the present state of medical knowledge. When the day comes that a cure or effective treatment is found for IBS, it is quite possible that these patients will find their anxiety diminishes, simply because their condition is now understood and treatable.

Stress and gut feelings

All of us notice a connection between fear, emotion, anxiety and how our insides behave, because there are direct nerve pathways between the brain and the intestines. That could explain why there are so many expressions in our language suggesting a link between the emotions and the gut. Consider this imaginary conversation between two women:

Anna: How did the promotion interview go?

Penny: Oh, fine in the end. I had real butterflies in my stomach all week, but I needn't have worried; I got the job.

Anna: That's wonderful news. I had a gut feeling that you would. What's John got to say about all the extra work you'll have to do?

Penny: Well, he's not too keen. Even now he keeps bellyaching whenever I have to work late. When I told him I'd been invited to apply for the job, I had an awful feeling in the pit of my stomach that he'd persuade me not to, but he didn't. Anyway, how are things with you? How's your new assistant?

Anna: He's doing fine. He's got real fire in his belly, and intends to get right to the top. The previous guy just didn't have the stomach for hard work. I kept on and on at him to work more effectively until he obviously thought I was a pain in the gut. Finally, when I'd really had a bellyful of him, I managed to get him promoted to Head Office!

Even a short snatch of conversation like this one contains eight phrases linking how we feel to how our insides feel. There are others too: It gets me right in the gut, He's got guts, My stomach turned over, Sick with worry, I can't stomach it . . . and probably many more. We certainly do connect our insides to our emotions.

As well as the usual brain-to-gut pathways, if you have IBS

you almost certainly have a bowel that over-reacts to *any* stimulus, whether to certain foods, or to being overloaded as in constipation, or to emotion.

A distressed mind can easily lead to an over-active colon (bowel). In research experiments, anger, anxiety and fear produced greater activity in the gut of IBS patients than it did in other people, possibly because IBS patients may have an unusually direct link between emotion and how the bowel works. It could be caused by the adrenalin that anger and anxiety produces; it could be that the bowel is extra-sensitive; but for some reason not yet fully understood if you have IBS you are more likely than other people to get digestive problems when you are upset.

When we are stressed, we tend to tense our muscles and restrict our breathing, and the body finds this stressful in itself. Relaxation techniques and breathing exercises can be helpful in calming down tense muscles, and, in the case of the abdominal muscles, making it less likely that they will go into spasm, and more likely that they will propel the food along in a calm smooth way causing neither diarrhoea nor constipation nor pain.

The vicious circle – and breaking it

Stress will always show itself somewhere – some people get migraine, some get asthma, others get one cold after another; we all have our own particular weak link, and for you it's your gut. When things are difficult for you, your bowel contracts more than other people's bowels do, causing pain; this pain is in itself stressful, making a vicious circle of stress-spasm-pain-stress.

Once something stressful has happened, your body remembers it, so that the next time that thing happens (or you think it might happen), your body's memory takes over and starts to produce adrenalin in anticipation of that event. Let's imagine that you had an argument with your neighbour. This is something particularly stressful, as we have to live cheek by jowl with our neighbours. During the argument your level of adrenalin will have risen, and your body will remember this. So next time you see your neighbour (or even think about him or her), the adrenalin will come rushing.in again, your insides will start to churn, and you start feeling stressed.

From now on, your aim must be to break this circle, and a good starting point is to look at what makes you feel stressed. Try looking at each area of your life in turn. The list that follows is of just a few ideas, but you will want to put in your own ones. Often it is helpful just acknowledging that something is stressing you, especially if up until now you haven't thought about it much, or perhaps have even denied it to yourself.

What makes me stressed?

At home

arguments with ....

jobs I have to do ....

jobs I'd like others to do or share ....

particular things about my husband/wife/partner ....
....

particular things about my children ....
....

particular things about my parents/in-laws ....
....

particular things about the people I live with ....
....

particular things about my neighbours ....
....

money worries ....

concern about my health, especially ....
....

concern about someone else's health, especially ....
....

sexual problems ....

too much to do ....

not enough to do ....

not being valued ....

anything else ....
....
....
....

At work
relationships with my boss ....
....
relationships with my colleague(s) ....
....
relationships with subordinates ....
....
relationships with others ....
....
lack of money ....
travelling ....
job insecurity ....
sexual harrassment ....
anything else (here you could look at the list on pages 73–4) ....
....
....
....

Other aspects of my life
leisure activities ....
....
my body/nose/ears/weight/hair ....
....
getting older ....
....
world events, especially ....
....
....
anything else ....
....
....
....

What makes my IBS worse?
eating out, because ....
....
going on holiday, because ....
....

meeting new people, because ....

....

worrying about ....

....

anticipating some things I have to do, especially ....

....

anything else ....

....

....

....

....

Write as frankly as you can, taking time to identify clearly those things that upset you, and particularly those things that make your IBS worse. Against each one write down what it is about *you* and what it is about *others* that causes the upset. Then write down one or two steps you could take to improve these things that worry you. If you don't do anything to improve things they might never improve. Later you can come back to this list and see how you can tackle some of these situations, and hopefully start to reduce the number of things that irritate your irritable bowel.

Having identified the things that upset you, or make you anxious or angry, write down against each one why you think this happens. Again, be honest with yourself. No one else will read this, but by being able to face up to the cause of the problem, you will be better able to manage it. Next, write down as many ideas you can think of for improving the situation – things you could do, things you could ask other people to do, ways in which you could seek help, ways in which you could alter your attitude to something – anything, in fact, which might make the situation easier for you to live with.

Only you know how stressful each of these is compared with the others, and what is a problem for one person may not be for another. However, you might be interested in a list that was published in 1967 in the *Journal of Psychosomatic Research* of the relative stresses of different events. It is known as the Holmes-Rahe Life Stress Inventory, and this is a very slightly adapted version of it:

Life Stress Inventory

Death of spouse	100
Divorce	73
Separation	65
Jail sentence	63
Death of close family member	63
Major personal injury or illness	53
Marriage	50
Being fired at work	47
Reconciliation with spouse or partner	45
Retirement	45
Major change in the health or behaviour of family member	44
Pregnancy	40
Sexual difficulties	39
Gaining new family member (e.g. birth, adoption, older child moving into the home, etc)	39
Major business readjustment (e.g. merger, reorganization, bankruptcy, etc)	39
Major change in financial state (much worse off or much better off)	38
Death of a close friend	37
Changing to a different line of work	36
Major change in the number of arguments with spouse (a lot more or a lot less)	35
Taking on a large loan (e.g. mortgage or business loan)	35
Foreclosure on mortgage or loan	30
Major change in responsibilities at work (e.g. promotion, demotion, job transfer)	29
Son or daughter leaving home	29
Trouble with in-laws	29
Outstanding personal achievement	28
Wife starts or ends work outside the home	26
Beginning or ending formal schooling	26
Major change in living conditions (better or worse)	25
Trouble with boss	23
Major change in working hours or conditions	20
Moving house	20
Moving to a new school	20
Major change in type or amount of recreational activities	19
Taking on a small loan (e.g. car or TV purchase)	17
Major change in sleeping habits	16
Major change in number of family get-togethers (more or less)	15
Major change in eating habits (e.g. more or less food, change in diet, change in times of eating)	15
Going on holiday	13
Christmas	12
Minor violations of the law (e.g. traffic offence)	11

Tick each of these life events that has happened to you during the last year, and add the total. A score of 150 or less shows you had relatively little life change, and so have a low susceptibility to stress-induced health breakdown. A score of 150–300 implies about a 50% chance of major health breakdown in the next two years. A score above 300 implies an 80% chance of major health breakdown in the next two years, according to the Holmes-Rahe statistical prediction model.

Many of these things are quite outside your control, but if you have learned how to cope with stress, and how to limit the amount of stress you have in other areas of your life, you have a much better chance of retaining your health.

4

Reduce Your Resistance to Stress

Reducing your resistance to stress is not at all the same thing as giving in to it. When you give in, your physical and mental health take a turn for the worse; when you reduce your resistance to it you should notice an improvement in your health in general and your IBS in particular.

Very few of us manage to avoid stress altogether. Therefore it becomes all the more important to reduce the level at which you start to feel stressed or anxious or angry, and the way your body and mind responds to it. If stress of a particular type or above a particular level triggers your IBS, then the more control you have over that, the better it is for your insides.

In the previous chapter, you wrote down those things that make you stressed, why you think this happens, and possibly some ways in which you might start to improve things. Look again at that list, and imagine one situation that upset you. Let's suppose it was an argument with your neighbour: as you remember it, your muscles will start to tense, your breath to become quicker and more shallow, your insides to churn. Now take a deep breath in and out, unclench your hands, lower your shoulders, relax your jaw, and breathe quietly and evenly. Imagine yourself seeing your neighbour next time and being quite calm. You are talking to him, but even if he is angry with you, your hands and shoulders are relaxed, and your breath is coming quietly and deeply. You are talking in a quiet calm voice. His anger is not getting to you. Continue to imagine yourself in control of this situation, feeling untroubled and inwardly quiet.

Try this with all the things on your list, starting with the ones that bother you least. See yourself feeling calm and quiet in situations that had bothered you only slightly, and when you know the method works, move on to more difficult ones. Allow yourself plenty of time for each, maybe tackling one each day or two. The important thing is to override your body's unpleasant memory of that situation. Some things may never completely resolve themselves, but if they can trouble you less than they did before you will feel better physically and emotionally.

We all have a limited ability to withstand stress, and people with IBS may have a more limited ability than some others. So don't waste the reserves you do have on pointless anger and hostility. If you do there will be nothing left when you need it.

One way to reduce unconstructive anger and anxiety is to cut down any negative 'self-talk'. Most of us talk to ourselves from time to time, some people more than others. What are you saying to yourself? And what effect is it having on you, and the tranquillity of your bowel? Are you reinforcing your anger, for example, by going over and over in your mind the argument with your neighbour, and all the things you'd like to say to him now you've had time to think about it? Or are you reinforcing a negative image you have of yourself: 'I can't do anything right', 'Life is so unfair to me', 'It must be my fault', 'I know that situation is going to make me anxious', and so on.

It doesn't need to be like that. You can replace these self-destructive thoughts with more positive ones that reduce your anger and anxiety, and make you feel better in yourself. (There is more on this in Chapter 9.)

The first thing to do is to stop each thought in its tracks – stone dead. As soon as you start to recall that argument, or anything else that arouses an unpleasant feeling in you – STOP. Just like that. End of thought. Consciously make your mind a complete blank for a few moments, and then fill it with a pleasant positive thought. Force yourself to do it. If you can't immediately think of a pleasant thought, recite a poem or a nursery rhyme, or sing a song – anything to cancel out those negative thoughts.

It is all too easy to dig a little groove for your mind, in which it instinctively grinds away with negative thoughts. And the deeper the groove, the harder it is to get out of it. So you have to recognize the moment it happens, and force yourself into thinking something pleasant and helpful. Before long you'll be surprised how seldom you think those useless thoughts; that groove will have disappeared, and you will be on the way to reducing the level at which things upset you.

Measure your resistance

You can measure your ability to cope with stress by completing the table below, which was developed by Lyle H. Miller and Alma Dell Smith of the University of Boston's Medical Center.

This test measures how much your way of life supports you and bolsters resistance to stress. Rate yourself for each of the 20 items on the scale from 1 (almost always) to 5 (never) according to how often they apply.
Add up your total score.

- *A score of 45 or less shows high resistance to stress and a healthy way of life;*
- *45 to 55 indicates that you may be susceptible to the effects of stress and could benefit from adjusting certain aspects of your daily life;*
- *over 55 and stress could be a serious risk, calling for a reappraisal of your general way of life.*

How much of the time are these statements true for you?

	Almost always	Most times	Some-times	Rarely	Never
1 My health is good (including eyesight, teeth, etc.)	1	2	3	4	5
2 My income meets my basic expenses	1	2	3	4	5
3 I am about the right weight for my build and height	1	2	3	4	5
4 I give and receive affection regularly	1	2	3	4	5
5 I express my feelings when angry or worried	1	2	3	4	5

	Almost always	Most times	Some-times	Rarely	Never
6 I have fewer than three caffeine-containing drinks (coffee, cocoa or cola) a day	1	2	3	4	5
7 I take part in regular social activities	1	2	3	4	5
8 I eat at least one full, well-balanced meal a day	1	2	3	4	5
9 I do something just for pleasure at least once a week	1	2	3	4	5
10 There is at least one relative within 50 miles (80 km) of home on whom I can rely	1	2	3	4	5
11 I have some time alone during the day	1	2	3	4	5
12 I get seven or eight hours of sleep at least four nights a week	1	2	3	4	5
13 My religious beliefs give me strength	1	2	3	4	5
14 I exercise hard enough to work up a sweat at least twice a week	1	2	3	4	5
15 I have a network of friends and acquaintances	1	2	3	4	5
16 I discuss problems such as housework and money with other members of the household	1	2	3	4	5
17 I have at least one friend I can talk to about personal affairs	1	2	3	4	5

18 I smoke no more than 10 cigarettes a day	1	2	3	4	5
19 I organize my time well	1	2	3	4	5
20 I have fewer than five alcoholic drinks a week	1	2	3	4	5

It's unlikely that you will score well on every single one, so try to work on those things you can control. For example, you may not be able to do much about the fact that you have no relatives within 50 miles, or that you have no religious beliefs, or don't enjoy taking exercise. But you could compensate by working on as many as possible of the other ones, even if you hadn't thought about them before. Perhaps you could make time alone for yourself each day, or consciously try to show more affection to friends and family, or discuss your problems with someone, or do something just for pleasure at least once a week.

Develop your resistance to stress

The ideas that follow are taken from my earlier books, *Coping Successfully with Your Irritable Bowel* and *Sleep Like a Dream – The Drug-Free Way* (Sheldon 1988), and if you can follow at least some of them you will start to reduce your resistance to stress:

- Develop a hobby that is relaxing and non-competitive. Give time to it.
- Several times a day, pause and do nothing. 'Sometimes I sits and thinks, and sometimes I just sits'.
- Try to arrange your home so that it is a place of peace and contentment. Look again at those things that reinforce a rushed and hurried life – the instant food, the breakfast bar where you perch as you bolt each meal, the high-performance car that encourages you to do 0–60 mph in no time at all, clocks in every room as a constant reminder of what time it is, the mobile phone in the garden so that you can be instantly in touch with your workplace . . . Slow down. Relax.
- Reconsider your view of stress in general. You may welcome it as a sign to everyone that your life is dynamic and complex,

or resent it as a sign of weakness. Either way it isn't doing your irritable bowel any good. It might help if you could accept it without any sense of pride or blame, yet resolve to reduce it in the interest of peaceful intestines.

- Maintain a balance of work and family time and responsibilities. Try not to let one area of your life dominate the others.
- Share the decision-making. You'll be amazed how well other people can cope if you trust them to.
- Consider taking a course in stress management. You will probably learn to: reduce the level at which you start to feel angry or anxious, recognize what triggers tension in you and how to prevent it, change how you look at different situations so you no longer see them as threatening, and start to feel hopeful about your condition.
- Smile at people as often as possible, whether you know them or not. It is difficult to keep an angry or unpleasant thought in your mind when you are smiling.
- Write down how you feel – especially if you feel angry. Write in great detail, even those things you find painful to write. Then tear it all up; don't leave it lying around for someone else to see or for you to dwell on. When you are angry or upset, the thoughts can completely fill your mind, making it difficult to concentrate on anything else. By writing it down you make 'space' in your head for more useful thoughts – in much the same way as the STOP method of coping with negative thoughts.
- Change your expectation of how someone will behave. Stress is often caused because we want someone to behave in a particular way, and s/he behaves completely differently. You will feel better if you can adjust your expectations.
- Look at those situations which you cannot change for the time being. Try to work out how you can learn to live with them in a way that won't make you stressed. Perhaps by removing some of the changeable problems you will have more resources to cope with those you can't change.
- Indulge yourself sometimes, without feeling that indulgence is wicked. Enjoy it.

- Make a list of those things that help you to wind down and relax. Here are some ideas to get you started, but you will be able to add many more of your own:

Relaxing activity	How often I do it	How often I'd like to do it
Watching TV	....	....
Soaking in a bath	....	....
Listening to music	....	....
Reading	....	....
Going for a walk	....	....
Talking to a friend	....	....
Fishing	....	....
Swimming	....	....
Playing a sport	....	....
Gardening	....	....
Going to the pub	....	....
Lying in the sun	....	....
Playing with the children	....	....
DIY	....	....
Cleaning the house	....	....
Getting out of the house	....	....
Jogging	....	....
Sleeping	....	....
Having your hair done	....	....
Playing an instrument	....	....
Writing letters	....	....
Just being by yourself	....	....
Cooking	....	....
Painting	....	....
Walking the dog	....	....
....	....	....
....	....	....
....	....	....

Against each item write down how often you do it, and then

how often you would *like* to do it. If there is a significant difference between these two factors, write down why that might be, and then what you might be able to do about it. What arrangements could be made? Who could help you? When could you start doing this?

For your general health, and for your IBS, you should put time aside regularly to do those things that relax you. This isn't something that should be dismissed as not all that important, something that you will get down to one day. If you are not getting enough opportunities to do these pleasurable things, start thinking what you could do *today* to make some changes.

5

Stress in Children

Spend a few minutes writing down on a piece of paper every word that describes you, both good and bad. The list might include such uncomplimentary descriptions as 'stupid', 'selfish', 'uncoordinated', 'not academic', 'fat', or 'gawky'. Then put a tick against any word that was used by your parents or teachers to describe you. You may be surprised to see how many unhelpful descriptions of yourself you are carrying around from your childhood.

Are you doing the same thing to your children? Are you perhaps unwittingly turning them into vulnerable or aggressive people by the way you treat them? Are you lowering their self-esteem, and thereby making them less able to cope with life, more prone to stress, more likely to get a stress-related condition like IBS?

Would you recognize stress in your child? Early warning signs are:

- tiredness
- losing a sense of perspective
- finding it harder to concentrate
- oversensitive to criticism
- eating more, or less
- losing or gaining weight
- sleep problems
- nightmares
- becoming accident-prone
- biting nails, pulling hair, jiggling knees
- complaints of frequent abdominal pain

Of course, any of these can be just part of the normal process of adolescence, and nothing particular to worry about. But most parents have an in-built sense of knowing when something is wrong, so listen to your inner voice, and try to help your children if you think they are particularly stressed.

Encourage them to eat balanced meals at reasonable times, sitting comfortably, and allowing plenty of time.

Take any bowel or digestive problem seriously; get it diagnosed by a doctor, but don't turn it into a momentous world issue. Show you care, but without encouraging the child to use constipation or indigestion as a manipulative tool. Try not to reward days off school with 'tummy ache' with presents, special food or treats.

Be aware of how your child sees himself in relation to others, what he is proud or ashamed of, in what ways he would like to be different. If he feels he is failing to live up to your expectations, he may become stressed. Maybe you could revise those expectations to fit in with how things really are.

Many children have false images of themselves, and focus on minor defects which other people just don't notice – a few spots, ears that stick out, crooked teeth. Encourage him to feel comfortable with himself as he is.

If he feels it is important to have lots of friends, to get invited to parties and discos, to enjoy the latest pop songs, or be good at sport his self-esteem will suffer if he isn't like that. A girl may envy a friend who has fair hair, blue eyes, a clear complexion and a good figure, while not appreciating that the friend may be bitchy, unkind and untruthful, while she herself is kind, thoughtful and well thought of. But she doesn't value these things in herself, and so has a quite unjustifiably low self-esteem.

These are things that parents can help children with. If you bring up your child to believe academic achievement or a good complexion is very important, yet your daughter is not very bright or has spots, her self-esteem will suffer, and will not improve just because she is in the school netball team unless you and she believe this is a high achievement.

Adolescents are easily deflated by criticism, by body image, by physical imperfections. Depending on how these feelings are handled, they could become shy and withdrawn, or aggressive and hostile. Try to be aware of the long-term effects your comments and off-the-cuff statements can have on your children and how they view themselves.

If your son says 'I failed the maths test', a reply such as 'I've always told you you were no good at maths' will simply reinforce his belief that he's no good. Instead you could say 'Well, I know you weren't feeling too good that day', or 'Why not ask your teacher for extra help with simultaneous equations/vectors/ Pythagoras, so that you'll pass next time?' If your daughter says, 'Everyone hates me', try a reply such as 'You had an argument with Jane today because. . . , but Sally and Anna are still good friends'. When she says, 'These jeans are a bit tight', replying 'Oh, you're just fat' will wither any self-esteem she might have. Instead, you could reply 'You are a bit overweight, but so are several other people in your class, and if you took a bit more exercise and ate more carefully you could easily lose some weight'.

IBS is not hereditary (i.e. it is not something you inherit in your genes), but it does tend to run in families. This could be because families tend to eat much the same sort of diet, or handle constipation wrongly, or be unaware of ways of handling stress. If you suspect that one of your children is under stress, take it seriously, and look at how your own feelings and attitudes might have contributed to it.

One-third of all adults with IBS have had the symptoms since childhood. Perhaps you could look back on your own childhood and see what triggered it; and then look at your children and see what you can do to prevent the same thing happening to them.

6

How to Relax

Imagine you are holding a lemon. Now, in your mind, cut it in quarters, and suck the juice of the whole quarter. Feel the juice on your lips and tongue, notice its sharpness. Did anything happen? You probably noticed saliva coming into your mouth, and your tongue reacting as if you really had felt the sharp tang of the lemon.

This is a simple example of how what goes on in the mind affects how the body responds. In irritable bowel syndrome the effect can be just as noticeable: you feel tense and anxious, and your intestines start going into spasm; you relax, and they calm down again. Perhaps one day researchers will identify the exact process by which this happens, and will develop a reliable treatment, but until then the best thing you can do for yourself is to remain as calm as possible, and avoid the sort of situations that provoke your intestines to make your life uncomfortable.

This chapter suggests several ways in which you can put the busy world to one side for a while and just r-e-l-a-x. (Another simple and relaxing exercise is described in a later chapter; see page 66.)

If you do not already make regular times for yourself in which to do nothing particular, this may not seem an easy or proper thing to do. From childhood we are encouraged to fill each moment with something worthwhile; doing nothing is 'lazy'. Some children were even taught to believe it is sinful. So we grow up unable to truly relax, and to feel guilty if we take time out for ourselves. How often have you been sitting quietly reading the paper or watching television or just putting your feet up, when your neighbour comes round. What do you do? The chances are that you apologize – 'I'm sorry, I was just sitting down for a moment while the kettle boiled/the paint dried . . .' and so on. The implication is that normally you would have been filling each moment with something wonderfully useful, and that you feel slightly guilty to be discovered doing something like putting your feet up for a few minutes.

In case these sort of feelings worry you, start by taking out only a few minutes each day for relaxing. Keep it short, just long enough to start feeling quiet inside yourself. Some very tense people find it extremely difficult to let go, and this is where *allowing* yourself to relax is much more effective than *making* yourself relax. Relaxation is about 'not going', and this is what so many people find difficult. So try to put aside those exhortations from childhood, and give yourself permission to be 'not doing'. You may have a lot of things to do, but however busy you are you can still spare a few minutes to sit quietly, and empty your mind of the pressures of the moment.

Learning to relax and let go has many benefits:

- you gain control over your life;
- an enhanced sense of well-being;
- you will feel more positive about yourself and your capabilities;
- you will become less anxious, more confident;
- you will be able to see the stresses in your life more in perspective;
- improved sleep
- a quieter digestive system
- a reduction in other stress-related conditions
- less fatigue
- your calmness may calm someone else who is upset or anxious

With a relaxation programme, you are in control. You are choosing to do it, and you can stop any time you want to. You can do as much or as little as you choose, when you choose, how you choose. You choose the position that suits you best, the time, the place, the exercises, and when you have had enough you choose to stop.

Some exercises will work for you, and perhaps some won't; some may not work at first, but will after a while. So try any that appeal to you, and come back to others later if you want to. While you are doing any form of relaxation, suspend all value judgements and intellectual criticism. And when you have finished, don't say to yourself, 'Well, I've done my relaxation for today', and then rush around as tense and stressed as ever, undoing all the good you have achieved.

Time and place?

Relaxation needs no special equipment, no skilled teacher or any other person, and no drugs. You can do it almost anywhere, it is simple, and it works.

What you do need is commitment to doing it, a reasonably quiet environment, a comfortable position, and a passive receptive attitude. If you can put aside a regular time each day it will be more effective, but even if you can't you will still benefit.

Where?

A quiet, warm, comfortable place is the ideal, but anywhere is better than nowhere. Try to be undisturbed by people or the telephone. Because you can relax lying or sitting, you will need either some floor space, or an upright or easy chair, or a sofa or meditation stool – whatever is convenient and comfortable.

When?

The best time is when you know you can put aside a few minutes and will be undisturbed. It may be first thing in the morning, or during the lunch break, or after work, or during the afternoon, or at bedtime. Try different times, and see which works best for you. Straight after meals seems to be a less good time for most people (because digestion seems to interfere with relaxation) but it may be just right for you. At least to begin with, you may settle down more quickly if you can choose the same time and place each day, so that you come to associate that time and place with being relaxed.

How long for?

Once you are doing some form of relaxation regularly each day or so, you will probably be taking somewhere between 15 and 30 minutes. It may be all at one time, or in two separate sessions, but the greatest gains will come if you can do it regularly. If you are saying to yourself, 'Where am I going to find an extra 30 minutes a day? I'm far too busy already', then that just demonstrates your need to relax. The time to relax is when you have no time to relax! If time is a problem to you, start with just five minutes once or twice a day, and build up when you feel able to – but do try to do at least something every day.

What do I wear?

What you wear is up to you. Whatever you are wearing right now will do. Or something completely different. If possible, have clothing that is loose around the neck and waist, but if you have no choice but to do relaxation exercises in a suit and tie, then just loosen anything that feels tight. If possible take off your shoes, and glasses if you wear them.

What position should I be in?

Simple answer – however you are most comfortable. Here are some ideas:

A. Sit on an upright chair with your spine straight. Keep your head easily balanced on your neck, with your chin pointing slightly down rather than slightly up. Imagine you are being pulled up like a puppet by a thread attached to the crown of your head (the crown is considerably further back than the forehead). Place your feet flat on the floor, legs slightly apart, hands resting comfortably on your lap, palms facing up or down whichever you prefer. If your feet don't touch the floor, rest them on a book or something similar. Keep your body equally balanced between the left and right side, rather than putting your weight and balance mainly on to one side. Move around until you feel symmetrical. Shut your eyes.

B. Sit in an easy chair, with your back resting comfortably against the back of the chair. A small cushion in the small of your back may give you more spinal support. Place your feet flat on the floor, a comfortable distance apart, and rest your hands on your lap, palms facing up or down. Shut your eyes.

C. Sit on a meditation stool, or a cushion, with your spine

straight, head pulled up from the crown, hands on your lap, eyes closed.

D. Lie on a sofa, with your body in a straight line, not twisted to one side or the other (see illustration). Your legs should be about shoulder-width apart, feet flopping outwards. Your hands can be by your side, or on your abdomen, palms facing up or down. You may be more comfortable if you put a small cushion or pillow under your head, or behind your knees, or in the small of your back. Shut your eyes.

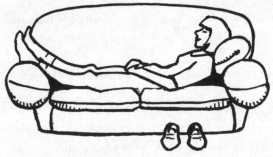

E. Lie on the floor on a thick blanket, in the same position as on a sofa.

These are all comfortable positions, and ideal for relaxing. But (unless you are relaxing specifically to help insomnia) the idea isn't to go to sleep, but rather to achieve deep relaxation while you are still awake. So lying on a bed is not ideal.

How do I finish?

When you have done as much as you want to, just remain where you are for a minute or two with your eyes closed, breathing quietly. Then open your eyes, and bring your mind back to the room you are in. Stretch your body from your heels to the top of your head, and if you are lying down, turn on to your side for a while. Then when you are ready, get up slowly. Don't rush off in a stressed hectic manner, as this will negate what you have done; instead, get up quietly and try to maintain a feeling of calm for as long as possible.

Now try the following exercises. At first nothing may seem to happen, you may be disappointed, and feel this is for other people but not for you. But don't be discouraged, because regular relaxation will be helping you even if you are unaware of it. Some people give up when they don't see instant results, but this is a pity because benefits begin before you are aware of any improvement.

Exercises for relaxation

There are numerous books available on how to relax, and your library or bookshop will probably have several. Included here is a collection of different forms of relaxation exercises, so you can choose which suits you best.

Exercises to relax your muscles

Exercise One: Do the exercise on page 66 – an easy way to relax wherever you are.

Exercise Two: Examine each part of your body in turn, and see if any set of muscles is tense. Work upwards from your toes to your head, thinking about each bit of you: your right foot, right leg, left foot, left leg – are they quite relaxed? Then your right hand, right arm, left hand, left arm – is there any tension there, particularly in your fingers? Now your abdomen – the source of your irritable bowel syndrome. Feel it being quite calm and relaxed, no tension, no spasm, just rising and falling gently as you breathe. Next your shoulders and neck, relaxed and heavy. Finally your jaw, mouth, eyes, forehead – no tension at all here, quite slack.

Tense people block out signs of tense muscles, so they become less aware of stress within themselves. A simple exercise like this can encourage you to be aware of tension in yourself, and so overcome it. As you notice any tense muscles, concentrate more on relaxing that set.

Exercise Three: To relax your shoulders, sit upright on a chair, hands relaxed in your lap and with your back straight but not stiff. Breathe in, and as you do so, raise your shoulders towards your ears. Hold for a count of 5, then slowly release your breath and lower your shoulders. Repeat a few times. This is a good exercise to do when you are stuck in a traffic jam.

Exercise Four: Sit or lie in a comfortable position. Close your eyes, and become aware of your breathing. Each time you exhale notice a different part of your body in turn and feel it being physically supported by the chair, sofa or floor. Become very aware of that part of you on each out-breath, and feel the heaviness of it. As you concentrate on it, say 'my [right foot] is warm and soft and heavy'. Imagine that foot sinking deeply into the floor or the sofa, so heavy that you couldn't possibly lift it up. Continue upwards until each part of you feels beautifully warm and soft and heavy.

Exercise Five: Having relaxed all your muscles in turn, you could now go one step further, and consciously tense them up. Once again, sit or lie in a comfortable position, and, starting with your feet, tense each set of muscles, then tense them even harder, then relax them. This tension will bring even greater relaxation. However, don't tense your abdominal muscles – they tense up all too easily, and any extra tension might make them worse.

Exercises with breathing

Breathing exercises are one of the easiest ways to achieve a feeling of calm, and they have the advantage that you can do them anywhere, at any time. They have the apparently contradictory effect of giving you energy when you feel tired, and calming you down when you feel tense. So next time you feel the need of a cup of coffee, or a cigarette, or a strong drink, just do breathing exercises for a minute or two instead – it's much better for your IBS.

When you are calm and relaxed you breathe from the diaphragm. Look at someone sleeping on his back, and you will see a gentle rising and falling movement from the area below the ribs. When you are tense you breathe from high up in your chest. So a quiet state of mind produces breathing from the diaphragm; but you can also put the cart before the horse and induce a state of calm by breathing from the diaphragm.

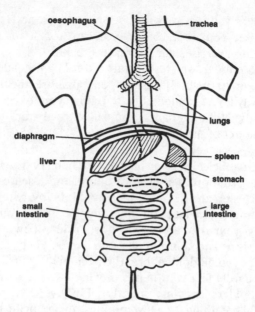

There is also another advantage in this level of breathing: the diaphragm is a strong sheet of muscle that separates the chest cavity from the abdomen (see illustration), and as it contracts during breathing it pushes the abdominal organs downwards and forwards, gently compressing and massaging them. So by doing breathing exercises regularly you benefit both your mind and your abdomen.

While you are doing the exercises, concentrate on your breath, and try not to let other thoughts come into your mind. If they do, don't get bothered or distracted by them, simply put those thoughts to one side for the moment and return your mind to your breath.

A word about breathing exercises

Sometimes this form of relaxation may bring to the surface of your mind thoughts and feelings that have been buried for a long time, and these thoughts may upset you. If this happens, be aware of them, accept them, and try not to become upset by them. Most thoughts of this kind are better out then in, but if they distress you just stretch, open your eyes, and come out of the exercise. You are in charge, you can stop at any time.

Breathing exercises can increase the level of oxygen in the blood to a point at which you start to feel light-headed, or your fingers begin to tingle. If this happens, just breathe in a panting shallow way for a few moments, to reduce your oxygen level. As with any unhelpful thoughts, you can stop any time you choose by coming out of the exercise.

Exercise Six: Start by doing an exercise lying on your back, with your feet a comfortable distance apart, and a sense of balance between the left and right sides of your body; move until you feel quite symmetrical. Place your hands in the area of your abdomen just below your ribs, and breathe from deep down so you feel that area rising and falling under your hands. Then, keeping your hands over your abdomen, breathe from high up in your chest so that you hardly feel your hands moving at all, but are aware of your shoulders moving slightly. Finally, return to quiet abdominal breathing for a few minutes, just noticing the rise and fall of your hands. When you are ready, get up slowly.

Exercise Seven: Lie as for Exercise Six, but place one hand on your abdomen as before, and one hand on your chest. As you breathe, notice which hand is moving, and by how much. Concentrate on the rise and fall of your hands. Then with the next breath, be aware of the air filling up from the diaphragm to the chest, of your lower hand moving before your upper one. Do this for a few minutes, all the time being aware of the air coming in through your nostrils and filling your lungs from the bottom up, and then of emptying again. Try to think of nothing but your breath coming in and out.

Exercise Eight: These next exercises can be done sitting or lying down. Find a comfortable position, shut your eyes, and be aware of breathing out. Notice how, after an out-breath, the in-breath just seems to happen. Again, do a long out-breath. Repeat several times: – long out-breath followed by a short in-breath – concentrating particularly on the out-breath.

Exercise Nine: This time, instead of noticing in-breaths separate from out-breaths, see them as one complete circular movement, in which each leads on from the other with no perceptible difference between them.

Exercise Ten: (1) breathe *out* deeply to get rid of stale air; (2) breathe *in* slowly and deeply to a count of *two*; (3) hold your breath for a count of *four*; (4) breathe *out* for a count of *four*. i.e. *in* two – *hold* four – *out* four. Do this for two or three minutes, but stop if you feel dizzy. All the time concentrate on the breath.

Exercise Eleven (alternate nostril breathing): First, identify your fingers – working outwards from the thumb they are the thumb, index finger, middle finger, ring finger, little finger.

Next; sit with your spine straight, eyes shut, and all your body relaxed. If you wear glasses it is best to remove them. (1) Place the index and middle fingers of your right hand on the bridge of your nose between your eyebrows. (2) With the ring finger of your right hand close the left nostril. (see illustration). If you are left-handed, you may prefer to reverse the instructions. (3) Breathe *out* through your right nostril, then breathe *in* through the same (right) nostril. (4) Lift your ring finger slightly and close your right nostril with your thumb, and breathe *out* through your left nostril, then *in* through the same (left) nostril. (5) Lift your thumb slightly and repeat from (2) for several minutes, remembering to breathe *out* first through each nostril. Listen to your

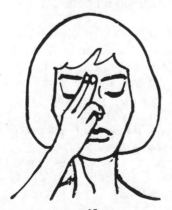

breathing. Concentrate on it. If your mind wanders, be aware of this, and bring it gently back.

Although this exercise seems complicated to describe, it is a simple soothing rhythm once you see how to do it. Gentle pressure on the nostrils is thought to relieve menstrual cramps, so there is a possibility that it might relieve abdominal cramps too.

Exercise Twelve: Get into a comfortable position. Relax all your muscles, and feel your body being supported by whatever you are sitting or lying on. Breathe naturally, and notice the cool breath coming in through your nostrils, and the warm air going out again. Be aware of this for a few minutes. Now, as you breathe out, visualize in any way that is comfortable to you the air carrying out from your body all the pain and tension that is inside you. Each breath takes away more pain and tension, and with successive breaths your whole abdominal area becomes relaxed and comfortable. When you are ready, stretch from your heels to the top of your head, open your eyes, and when you are ready get up.

Exercise Thirteen: This is reproduced from the Workers' Educational Association pack on Women and Health, with permission of the Health Education Authority. The most effective way to do this exercise is to record it on to tape, and play it back when you want to relax. Read it into the microphone using a slow calm voice; pause for a moment at the end of each phrase. If you are not happy with the first recording, make a note of any changes you need to make, and do it again.

Begin by breathing *out* first. Then breathe in easily, just as much as you need. Now breathe out slowly, with a slight sigh, like a balloon slowly deflating. Do this once more, slowly . . . breathe in . . . breathe out . . . and as you breathe out, feel the tension begin to drain away. Then go back to your ordinary breathing, even, quiet, steady.

Now direct your thoughts to each part of your body in turn, to the muscles and joints.

Think first about your left foot. Your toes are still. Your foot feels heavy on the floor. Let your foot and toes start to feel completely relaxed.

Now think about your right foot . . . toes . . . ankles . . . they are resting heavily on the floor. Let both your feet, your toes, ankles start to relax.

Now think about your legs. Let your legs feel completely relaxed and heavy on the chair. Your thighs, your knees roll outwards when they relax, so let them go.

Think now about your back, and your spine. Let the tension drain away from your back, and from your spine. Notice your breathing, and each time you breathe out, relax your back and spine a little more.

Let your abdominal muscles become soft and loose. There's no need to hold your stomach in tight. It rises and falls as you breathe quietly – feel that your stomach is completely relaxed.

No tension in your chest. Let your breathing be slow and easy, and each time you breathe out, let go a little more.

Think now about the fingers of your left hand – they are curved, limp and quite still. Now the fingers of your right hand . . . relaxed . . . soft and still. Let this feeling of relaxation spread – up to your arms . . . feel the heaviness in your arms – up to your shoulders . . . let your shoulders relax, let them drop easily . . . and then let them drop even further than you thought they could.

Think about your neck. Feel the tension melt away from your neck and shoulders. Each time you breathe out, relax your neck a little more.

Now, before going any further, just check to see if all these parts of your body are still relaxed – your feet, legs, back and spine, tummy, hands, arms, neck and shoulders. Keep your breathing gentle and easy. Every time you breathe out, relax a little more, and let all the tensions ease away from your body. No tensions . . . just enjoy this feeling of relaxation.

Now think about your face. Let the expression come off your face. Smooth out your brow and let your forehead feel wide, and relaxed. Let your eyebrows drop gently. There's no tension round your eyes . . . your eyelids slightly closed, your eyes are still. Let your jaw unwind . . . teeth slightly apart as your jaw unwinds more and more.

Feel the relief of letting go.

Now think about your tongue, and throat. Let your tongue drop down to the bottom of your mouth and relax completely. Relax your tongue and throat. And your lips . . . lightly together, no pressure between them.

Let all the muscles in your face unwind and let go – there's no tension in your face – just let it relax more and more.

Now, instead of thinking about yourself in parts, feel the all-over sensation of letting go, of quiet and of rest. Check to see if you are still relaxed. Stay like this for a few moments, and listen to your breathing . . . in . . . and out . . . let your body become looser, heavier, each time you breathe out.

Now continue for a little longer, and enjoy this time for relaxation.

Finally, wriggle your hands a little, and your feet. When you are ready, open your eyes and sit quietly for a while. Stretch . . . then slowly start to move again.

Practise some form of relaxation every day, in the car, at a computer, at the sink, ironing board, workbench, desk . . . wherever you are. Just pause, take a deep breath, and consciously relax your muscles. Once you have practised being relaxed in a calm place on your own, you will be able to be relaxed at other times – in a meeting, during discussions, while driving, shopping, doing household jobs, when you are bored or frustrated, and even when your spouse or children drive you mad. Having developed the habit of relaxation, it will come quite naturally to you.

In the early days, when you have achieved a state of peacefulness even for a few minutes, take time to mentally record the experience. Recall what you did, how you felt, and remember yourself in that situation being relaxed. This will reinforce your expectation of being relaxed, and it will get steadily easier.

As you go through the day, notice how you are standing or sitting. If you are standing with your weight on one leg, move until both feet are carrying equal weight. When you sit with your legs crossed, become aware of it, and place both feet flat on the floor with your legs relaxed. (If, like me, you are fairly short, this is easier said than done, as most chairs seem to be designed for tall people with long legs!) Are your shoulders tense? Then lower them, feel your neck stretching out, your muscles relaxed. Are you tapping your fingers, banging your knees, clenching your teeth, jingling the coins in your pocket? Notice it, then just relax those tense muscles. Get into the habit of noticing these little things about you during the day, and making changes. The build-up of tension in your muscles is a sign of your tense mind; and by relaxing muscles that you can see and control, you will be aware of the general tension in your body that is also present in your abdomen. You have no direct control over the muscles of the colon (bowel), but the tension within you affects the way those muscles propel food; reducing your overall level of stress and tension will indirectly cause those muscles to relax.

7

Meditation and Yoga

Mantras, joss sticks, and standing on your head – is this your image of meditation and yoga? A load of Eastern nonsense? All very well for people who like that kind of thing, but not for you?

Mantras are words said repetitively to help concentrate the mind and direct it away from the present. In your life you may achieve a similar effect by concentrating so hard on something that the effort becomes quite relaxing.

Standing on your head is a form of exercise that also takes up all your concentration, and leaves you feeling relaxed and invigorated. You may be taking exercise that has a similar effect.

So these disciplines are perhaps not so wildly different from what you already do. But meditation and yoga can achieve other benefits that most ordinary forms of exercise can't. Regularly practising either of these can lower your heartbeat and blood pressure, improve your sleep, decrease anxiety, increase alertness, ability to concentrate and general well-being, as well as bringing a feeling of calm and release from tension.

People who practise meditation regularly are less anxious than others, less prone to stress, and recover quicker after stressful incidents.

If you think it may be worth trying, this chapter has some ideas for simple meditation exercises. You may recognize some of them from *Coping Successfully with Your Irritable Bowel* (Sheldon, 1988), but there are also some new ones.

Meditation

As with all relaxation exercises, meditation can be done anywhere, but it is more beneficial if you can choose a time and place where you will be comfortable and undisturbed. It is important to divert your mind from your normal thought processes. Suspend all judgement, and intellectual criticism. Just be patient and passive, and in time you will be pleased at the changes you start to notice, both in your mind and, hopefully, in your irritable bowel.

Meditation, like breathing exercises, can sometimes bring thoughts to the surface of your mind that make you feel agitated or anxious. This is quite normal. If this happens, simply open your eyes, have a good stretch, and come out of the exercise. As before, you are in control, you can stop when you want to.

Meditation exercises

Exercise One: As with the breathing exercises, sit or lie in a comfortable position. Take your mind over your whole body, and consciously relax all your muscles from your feet up to your head. Concentrate particularly on whatever part of your body you often tense up. Breathe normally. When you feel quite relaxed, as you breathe out say the word 'one' either out loud or to yourself. Then breathe in normally. Continue like this, saying 'one' each time you breathe out. Try to concentrate on the normal breathing and the word 'one'. Your mind will probably wander, and if it does just be aware of this and bring your thoughts gently back to the word 'one'. After about 10 minutes continue normal breathing without saying 'one', just being quiet, with your eyes closed. Then open your eyes, take in the room around you, and when you are ready get up. If you prefer, you could say 'peace' instead, or any word that seems right for you.

After each exercise don't worry whether you have successfully achieved what you believe meditation to be. In time it will come.

Exercise Two: This is an exercise in noticing yourself. As you sit quietly, notice your internal feelings: your breathing, any digestive rumbles, your closed eyelids on your eyeballs, your tongue in your mouth, your heart beating, your hands and feet resting against the floor or against a part of your body. Then notice other body feelings: your toes in your socks and shoes, the waistband of your trousers or skirt, your neckband or tie, your cuffs around your wrists, how your clothes feel on your skin. Finally notice external sounds: cars going by, dogs barking, someone walking past, people talking, any smells in the air. Identify each thing, but do not allow yourself to think about it or get distracted by it. Repeat this from the beginning as many times as you want to.

ExerciseThree: Place a lighted candle a few feet in front of you. Concentrate on it until you feel you can't look at it any longer. Then shut your eyes, and you will see the after-image of the candle and the flame in front of you. Concentrate on this after-image until it fades from your mind. Then open your eyes and look at the real candle again. Repeat this as many times as you want to.

Exercise Four: Create in your mind an image of your trouble-some gut (or any other part that's bothering you). How you see it can be abstract, or symbolic or anatomically correct – it doesn't matter. Just hold the picture in your mind. Now imagine your body's defence mechanisms (again this can be abstract or symbolic or anatomically correct) moving to your gut, soothing it, calming it. Let your imagination run wild, see your gut responding, see any spasms dying down, any muscular contortions fading away. Now your gut is pain free, and propelling food in a smooth gentle way, up the right side of your abdomen, across the middle, and down the left side, like a river flowing. Visualize yourself going about your life with your bowel made pain-free by your body's natural mechanisms. Then open your eyes, observe the room you are in, take a few breaths, stretch, and get up slowly.

Exercise Five: As you breathe normally, focus your thoughts on the rise and fall of your abdomen, and of the air flowing in and out of your nostrils. As you breathe *in* count 1, and as you breathe *out* count 2, *in* count 3, *out* count 4, and so on up to 10. Then start again: *in* 1, *out* 2, *in* 3, *out* 4 . . . Don't attempt to control or manipulate your breath. Just let it happen naturally, being aware of it. Continue doing this as long as you want to, trying to keep your mind on nothing but your breathing.

Exercise Six: Hold five beads or pebbles in one hand. Pass them slowly one at a time to the other hand. Feel each one, count it, hear the sound it makes against the others. Pass the beads from one hand to the other as many times as you want to, focusing your attention on the beads, thinking of nothing else apart from them, their sound and feel.

Exercise Seven: This is a useful exercise if something is troubling you and preventing you giving your thoughts to other things. Sit comfortably, breathing quietly. Now focus on whatever is disturbing you, but without getting caught up in it. Don't allow yourself to wallow in worrying thoughts. Try to give a shape to this problem – any shape you like – until it is an actual *object*, not just a thought. Now imagine you are standing back from this object that is your worry, and you are looking at it objectively. In your imagination get a box and put the shape into it. Get some wrapping paper and sellotape and scissors, and use the scissors to cut out some wrapping paper, wrap it around the box, and secure it with sellotape. Take time being really imaginative about this. When the shape is nicely wrapped up in the box, take the box and put it somewhere safe where you can't see it while you get on with your life, but where it will be when you need to face up to it again. So now it is put away somewhere. Now see yourself getting on with your life with this particular problem out of the way. You can leave it there as long as you choose to, but at some time you will need to come back to it, to unwrap it and face it, although all the time you know you can put it back in its box when you want to. End the session by returning your thoughts to where you are at present, and the room you are in. As before, take a few breaths, stretch, and get up when you feel ready. Try to do this exercise with imagination and interest, without any sense of intellectual judgement about it; you will then be able to put worrying problems aside and get on with living your life more constructively.

Exercise Eight: This is reproduced from the Workers' Educational Association pack on Women and Health with permission of the Health Education Authority. Record it on to tape in a slow, calm voice, pausing slightly after each phrase:

Imagine yourself walking out of the room you are in. You go outside, and see a magic carpet there. You get on to the carpet and make yourself comfortable. You are going to fly right away from here to somewhere much warmer. You are flying above towns and villages, fields and farms. The houses and cars look unreal, like matchbox toys. Now you are over a beach, and now over the sea. At first the sea is grey, but as you get to a warmer climate it gets bluer and bluer. You can feel the sun beating down on you, warming you up.

Ahead you see a lush island with palm trees, white sands and clear blue sea. You land on the beach and look around you for a minute or two breathing in the richly scented warm air. You take a stroll on the beach barefoot, and feel the warmth of the sand on the soles of your feet. Dip your toes in the sea; it feels warm and refreshing.

Now walk into the jungle. There are beautiful exotic flowers everywhere – they smell wonderful and have clear bright colours – pinks, yellows, turquoise. High above you are monkeys jumping from tree to tree chattering to each other, and parrots flying around. Ahead you see a clearing through the trees, and you walk towards it. There is a sleepy green lagoon bathed in green light from the sun passing through the tallest palm trees. On the lagoon is a little dinghy, and you get into it and lie down.

You are bobbing gently in the lagoon in a pool of green light. You can hear the monkeys and birds in the jungle, but they sound a long way off. You can smell the fragrance of the exotic flowers and fruits. Just enough sun can get through the trees to warm your body as you lie on the dinghy. Let yourself completely unwind as you relax, taking in the warmth and smells and sounds of the jungle.

When you are ready to come back, get up from the dinghy, and walk slowly back through the jungle to your magic carpet. Make yourself comfortable on the carpet again for your journey home. You are flying over the sea, then over land, and now you can see your home town. You land back where you started from, and walk back into the room.

Yoga

All these meditation exercises have involved nothing more

strenuous than sitting in a chair or lying on the floor. Yoga postures are slightly more active. The best way to do yoga really is to join a class with a qualified instructor who will teach you to do the postures correctly. But if that isn't possible, here are some simple ones to start on.

Yoga exercises

The Corpse (see illustration): This is the most basic posture, and the one with which you should end every yoga session. Although it looks easy, you must concentrate to achieve the effect of calmness. Just lie on the floor, on a thick blanket if possible, making sure you are warm and comfortable. Draw your toes up towards you, stretching the heels, then relax your feet so that they flop out sideways. Place your arms a little way from your body, with the palms facing upwards (but if this is not comfortable, put your hands however suits you best). If necessary place a small cushion or pillow under your head or the small of your back. Make sure your body is straight and symmetrical between the left and right sides. Now consciously relax each group of muscles up your body, and remain like this for about 5 minutes. If you notice any distracting sounds, just say to yourself 'These sounds do not matter'.

(So yoga doesn't have to involve complicated lotus positions, and standing on your head!)

The Thunderbolt: This is another simple posture (see illustration). Sit back on your heels, hands resting on your knees, eyes looking straight ahead, with your head feeling as if it is being pulled up by a thread attached to the crown. If sitting on your heels is not very comfortable, try using a cushion or pillow to raise your buttocks slightly off the floor, and relieve tension in your knees and ankles. Or use a meditation stool if you have one. Focus your gaze on an object ahead of you and breathe evenly in and out for a few minutes. When you feel quite calm and peaceful, try:

The Lion: Remaining in the same position as for the Thunderbolt, open your eyes and mouth as wide as possible, stick your tongue out towards your chin, and give a loud ROAR! Doing this

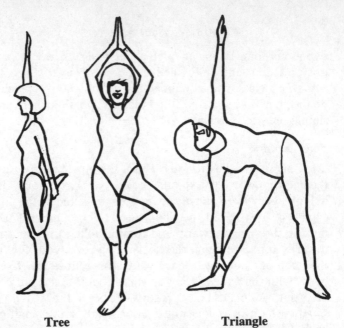

Tree
looking straight ahead

Triangle
looking at raised left hand and with
hand grasping ankle, or lower leg

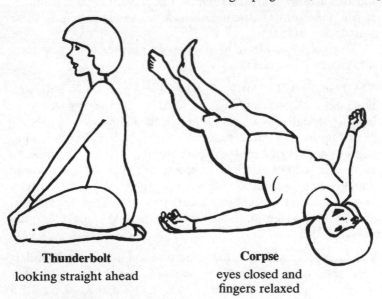

Thunderbolt
looking straight ahead

Corpse
eyes closed and
fingers relaxed

56

two or three times can bring a wonderful sense of relieving tension.

The Tree: This is another very relaxing posture, and much easier than it looks. There are several variations, and two are illustrated here. The sense of balance will probably come quickly, but to begin with you might feel more stable if you lean your back against a wall. It is easier to hold the position if your feet and legs are bare. Bend your right knee, and taking your right foot in both hands place it against the inside of your left knee, or higher if you can manage it. Press the sole of the right foot well into the left leg. Now, looking straight ahead, raise your hands above head, and place the palms together above your head. Hold this for as long as you feel comfortable, then repeat with the left foot against the right leg, and all the time looking straight ahead as far away as possible.

A variation is to raise the left leg behind you, holding it with your left hand, while raising your right arm. Then repeat the posture, holding your right leg behind you and raising your left arm. Again, look straight ahead all the time.

The Triangle (see illustration): Face forwards, legs wide apart, arms out sideways level with your shoulders. Turn your right foot out and your left foot in. Now bend to the right, sliding your right hand down your right leg until it reaches as far as it comfortably will; this may be flat on the floor, or to grasp your ankle, or placed against your knee. At this stage, only reach as far as you can easily. Without turning your hips look up at your left hand which should be raised vertically above you. Hold for as long as you can, then repeat, reversing the instructions to the left.

Salute to the Sun (see illustrations): This is an ancient Chinese exercise, traditionally done first thing in the morning to tone up the muscles and make you feel good for the day. It combines six yoga postures in a sequence of ten movements, and four of the positions are repeated. You might find it easier to remember the sequence if you can record it in a calm soothing voice, allowing short pauses between each movement.

This variation of Salute to the Sun is taken from *Yoga* by

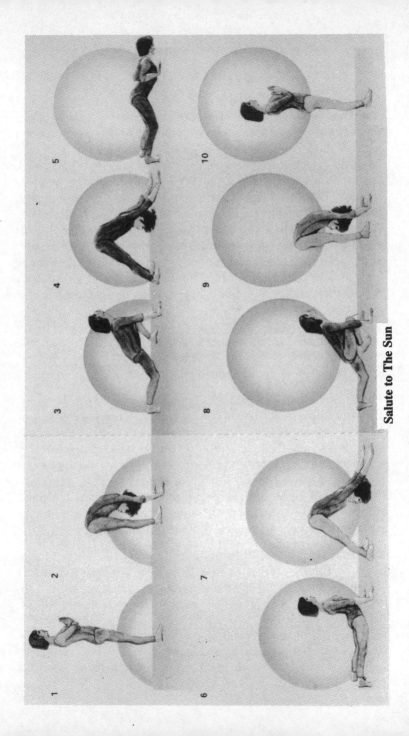

Salute to The Sun

Sophy Hoare, published by Macdonald. To begin with you might find it easier if you ignore the breathing instructions, and then include them when you feel more familiar with the routine.

1. Stand with your feet together, knees straight, back stretched up but not tense. Place the palms of your hands together in front of your chest and breathe in slowly and deeply. Breathe out as you move into the second position.

2. Bend forward from the hips until your hands are on the ground a short distance in front of you. Move your hands forward until your legs are straight. Tuck in your chin towards your chest, and pull your stomach in. Then breathe in as you move into the third position.

3. Keeping your hands and arms in the same place, stretch one foot as far as you can behind you, at the same time bending your other knee and bringing it forward between your arms, and lifting up your head and slightly arching your back. Breathe out as you move to the fourth position.

4. Take your other foot back level with the first and straighten both legs. Try to press your heels towards the ground. Drop your head down so that your chin is tucked into your chest. Keep your arms straight and try to flatten and extend your spine. Take another breath in, and breathe out as you go into the fifth position.

5. Keeping your hands and feet where they are, bend your arms and lower your body to the ground, touching the ground with your toes, knees, chest and forehead. Pull your stomach in as you breathe out.

6. As you breathe in, lift up your head and bend backwards, straightening your arms and legs so that the weight of your whole body is on your hands and toes.

7. As you breathe out, lift your bottom into the air, drop your head and tuck your chin in towards your chest, and straighten your legs. This is the same as position four.

8. As you breathe in, bring one leg forward so that the foot rests as nearly as possible between your hands. Look up and bend back as in position three. Breathe out fully as you move into position nine.

9. This is a repeat of position two. Bring the other foot forward next to the first. Straighten your legs and tuck your chin in.

10. Breathe in as you lift your hands off the ground and stand up with a straight back. Join the palms in front of your chest.

You can repeat the sequence as many times as you like, though it is best to start gradually.

8

Making Changes

Getting to know your insides

Curled up snugly inside your abdomen is approximately 30 feet (9 metres) of tubing called the bowel. The first 20 feet (6 metres) is called the small intestine, because it is small in diameter (about 1 inch / 3 cm). It is one enormous coil, roughly behind the umbilicus (belly button), and in it the food is broken down by digestive juices until it is liquid enough to be absorbed through the walls of the small intestine into the bloodstream so it can be carried away all round the body, to be used for making, building and repairing.

The food that is left moves on to the large intestine (called large because it is about 2½ inches / 6 cm in diameter), also known as the colon, and the source of much of your problem. The colon starts low down on the right hand side of the abdomen, and it is

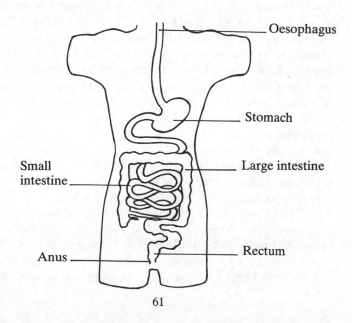

Oesophagus

Stomach

Small intestine

Large intestine

Anus

Rectum

here that the last stages of digestion are completed as the food moves up the right hand side of the abdomen, across the middle, and down the left hand side to the rectum. The remains of your last meal enter the colon as a semi-liquid mass, and the purpose of the colon is to absorb the water back into the body, and store any waste material until there is enough for it to be passed out of the body via the rectum and anus (back passage). By the time this waste material reaches the end of the large intestine it is quite compact, brown and fairly dry.

This waste matter is propelled through the large intestine by muscular waves called 'peristalsis', and it is the abnormal movement of the waves that cause cramping pains, constipation and diarrhoea. Tests have shown that in people with IBS, the gut (another name for the intestines) reacts more vigorously during anger, stress and anxiety than it does in people without IBS. So it's obviously in your best interests to keep your bowel happy, and running smoothly and placidly.

Your bowel is not your enemy, though you may think it is. It doesn't just lurk there in your abdomen waiting for an opportunity to embarrass you or cause you pain. Most of the time it works hard doing a monotonous job digesting one meal after another, moving one lot of food along to make way for the next, and maybe wishing you could make its role in life easier.

Instead, what do you do? You feed it food it doesn't like; other people's bowels happily digest onions or strawberries or coffee, but if yours doesn't then it will be happier if you don't expect it to. You deprive it of visits to the toilet; almost certainly your bowel will want to empty some of its contents soon after the first meal of the day (because nature has programmed it that way), but instead of allowing yourself time for this you bolt down a meal that could hardly be called breakfast, rush around grabbing briefcase, children, razor or mobile phone, so when by mid-morning you graciously allow yourself five minutes in the toilet your bowel has gone off the whole idea. And finally, knowing that your bowel likes a quiet life, you torture it with a whole range of unpleasant emotions that it really can't handle and which send it into a turmoil of spasm.

Take time to get to know your intestines – what they like, and most particularly what they don't like. Respect them, in the same way that you should respect your heart, your kidneys, even your feet. Your body has to last you for the whole of your life, so treat it well. You can't trade it in for a more beautiful, less troublesome model, so learn to live in peace with it and it will repay you well.

Many people's IBS started after going on a crash diet. Why did you feel the need to diet? Unless you are seriously overweight, learn to love your body for what it is, not for some stereotyped idea of what other people think it should be. Your body is your responsibility; don't blame yourself if it isn't exactly what you'd like it to be, but accept it, even learn to love it. For all its faults, you probably wouldn't really want to be in anyone else's.

Ignorance about our bodies can lead to feelings of embarrassment and powerlessness, especially in our relationships with doctors. The more you know about how your body works, the more you will feel in control of it, rather than the other way round. Find out as much as you can about irritable bowel syndrome, and any other condition you have, so that you are better able to take responsibility for your own health. It's not your fault that you have IBS, so don't feel guilty about it or allow others to make you feel guilty. It's all too easy to take on board the feelings of your doctor, your boss, members of your family, and feel you shouldn't have this condition because it inconveniences their lives. Put these feelings of guilt to one side and decide that from today onwards your whole approach to your IBS is going to be different, because from now on you are going to take responsibility for your own health.

Change: getting started

Today is the beginning of the rest of your life, and is as good a time as any to make some changes. No one can force change upon you, it has to be something you want to do for yourself, like stopping smoking or biting your nails. But as the saying goes, 'There's nothing quite so powerful as an idea whose time has come.' Perhaps you might decide that as from today you will:

- give up eating the food in the canteen because it doesn't agree with you;
- learn some simple relaxation techniques and practise them regularly;
- go jogging twice a week;
- not use swear words;
- tackle the problem of why other people leave the place in such a mess;
- explain to your wife that you want to change your job;
- explain to your husband that you'd like him to help more often with the washing up;
- make more time for yourself;
- learn Spanish/take up an instrument/start a new hobby;
- seek help for a particular problem.

Whatever it is, *you* have decided to make the change, *you* have taken responsibility for that aspect of your life, and *you* will make it succeed.

Start change in small doses, and in only one area of your life at once. When you feel unsure or anxious about the decision you've made, ask yourself:

- What's the worst thing that can happen?
- How likely is it to happen?
- What can I do to reduce the chance of it happening?

By thinking any change through you are much more likely to make a success of it. Define your goal in simple, active, positive words, as if you were saying them to a friend:

- I go jogging every day now
- My husband shares the washing up
- I put aside some time for myself every day
- I'm learning Spanish
- Saying NO is becoming much easier
- I have decided to look for a new job

Imagine yourself living with this new goal. Tell yourself, 'I can do it'.

Each time you manage to change something, reward yourself in some small way. Congratulate yourself on this achievement. It won't take long to realize that change is possible, and rewarding.

If making a change is going to be difficult, consider who can help you – friends, colleagues, any organizations. There's always someone out there who can give you the help and encouragement you're looking for. If you have tried before, and failed, think carefully about where you went wrong; see it in terms of a mistake *you* might have made (perhaps you chose the wrong time to ask, or used the wrong words, or the wrong tone of voice) and work out how you could do it differently this time. Practise the words until you feel comfortable with them; if necessary, try them out on a friend you can trust and see whether he or she thinks they sound right. If the situation was one that affected only you (like taking regular exercise or giving up smoking) acknowledge to yourself the real reason you didn't succeed on a previous occasion, and see if you can change it this time round.

We may not be able to change our basic personalities, but we can change our beliefs, expectations (of ourselves and of others), our goals, attitudes, the choice of words we use, and our body language. How many of these various characteristics that go to make up your personality are contributing to your irritable bowel syndrome, and to what extent could you change them if it meant a more peaceful digestive system? These are all things that you can take responsibility for, and you have the power to change them.

Managing change

You may now feel that it is both desirable and possible to make some changes and to reduce the stress in your life, if only because it will probably help your irritable bowel syndrome. From the previous chapters you will be able to recognize signs of stress in yourself, know what events are likely to make your IBS worse, and be able to acknowledge areas of your life that are less calm than they might be.

Maybe the time has now come when you think to yourself, 'Yes, there's probably something in all this. Perhaps I'll give it a whirl. It can't do any harm. It may even do some good. I wonder where I should start'.

You may have seen books on relaxation, yoga, or meditation, and quickly decided that they are not for you. They may be all right for people who like that kind of thing, but sitting in the lotus position or standing on your head or doing things with meditation beads is not the image you have of yourself.

Well, that's no problem, because one way of starting involves nothing more than just sitting – anywhere, any time – and it won't take long. You can do it in the train, on the bus, at your desk or workbench, at home. Wherever you are, you will look absolutely normal, but you will be starting to manage your irritable bowel.

So start by just sitting. Keep your spine straight, your eyes closed, your feet flat on the floor, and your hands loosely on your lap. For the next few minutes try to put to one side all those thoughts that are racing around in your head. You can come back to them soon enough – they'll still be there! Simply breathe in and out in your normal way. Think of nothing except your breath: what it feels like, the sound it makes, the cool breath coming into your nostrils, and the warm breath coming out again. Concentrate on your breathing. If your mind wanders, don't feel guilty about it, just bring your thoughts back to your breathing. Do this for a few minutes. When you feel ready to stop, just sit quietly for a moment or two then open your eyes, take in your surroundings, and get up slowly. That wasn't difficult, was it? You have now taken a few minutes out of your busy life to relax. You have made a start. Unlikely as it may seem, if you can do nothing more demanding than this a few times every day, you should begin to notice an improvement. When you feel comfortable with this simple breathing exercise, you may like to try some others from Chapter 6.

A similar exercise is useful when you feel things catching up on you. If you are facing a difficult situation, or someone says or does something that upsets you, try the following:

(1) Let your breath out, then breathe in, then do a long out-breath.

(2) Continue to breathe calmly while you lower your shoulders, relax your neck, and unclench your jaw and your hands.

(3) Try to keep your voice low and calm.

(4) Visualize your digestive system remaining calm and peaceful.

(5) Say to yourself, 'I am in control of this situation'.

At the end of each day, spend time relaxing. Recall each episode of the day where you felt things got on top of you, or you did not react as well as you would like to have done. Ask yourself, 'How could I have handled that better?' Think whether you have eaten inappropriately, or felt rushed or stressed: was it necessary, and how could you have avoided it? Resolve to make whatever changes will prevent the same things happening next time.

With any potentially stressful situation,

(a) PLAN IT: think in advance about how you will handle it, and what words you will use;

(b) DO IT: try to follow your plan;

(c) REVIEW IT: and afterwards analyse how it went, and if necessary how it could go better next time.

9

Planning for Change

How do you feel about change? Does it excite you? Do you dread it? Do you feel you'd like to change things but are afraid to? Or don't know how?

You could start by making an action plan. Things don't have to stay as they are. They can change, and *you* can be the one that makes the changes.

Get out a large sheet of paper, and on it draw a picture of your life as you would like it to be in two or three years' time. You could divide it into different areas, such as Home, Work, Leisure, etc. In each section draw the New You, as you would like to see yourself. Perhaps draw the sort of house you would like to live in, where you would like to be living, what possessions you would like to have (or to discard). Draw yourself in the type of job you would like to be doing, and where, and with whom. Write down words or phrases or sentences that describe what that area of your life will be like. Include all your deepest ambitions. Try to take at least half an hour on this, longer if possible. Be imaginative and free-thinking. Think widely and creatively. Don't be tied down by rational intellectual judgements. Say to yourself: 'If I really wanted to, I could be:

- running my own company
- living in Hawaii
- reconciled with John
- divorced
- a photographer
- teaching dry-stone-walling
- learning how to hang-glide
- feeling in control of my IBS'

Put down in words or pictures all the things you would like your life to contain, both possible and impossible. Then give yourself permission to want these things.

Now choose one or two that you really would like to be or have or do in the next twelve months: 'In a year from now I'd like to . . .'

Filling in the chart may help you.

What I hope to achieve by this time next year

....
....
....
....

What obstacles are preventing me doing this?

....
....
....
....
....

What am I afraid of?

....
....
....
....
....

What are my particular strengths to achieve this?

....
....
....
....
....

Who could help me? Who could I talk to? Who knows how to do it?

....
....
....
....

What further information do I need to be able to do this?

....
....
....
....

Where is help and advice available?

....
....
....
....

In order to do this, my first step will be:

....
....
....
....

Having got this far, now go ahead and take that first step – today if possible. Don't say, 'But I can't, because . . .' – that way lie negative thoughts and dead-ends and frustration. Try to break down those things that are standing in the way of your goal, and build up those things that will allow it to happen.

Your job

One area of people's lives that seems to cry out for change is their employment. To become employed rather than unemployed; self-employed rather than work for someone else, or the other way round; to work shorter or longer hours; to have more or less responsibility, more or less pressure; to work in a different area or environment, or with different people; to do the same thing, but differently; or to do something totally, entirely, mind-bendingly different.

More working days are lost each year from stress-related illnesses than from the common cold, and in the majority of cases the job itself is the cause of the stress.

It could be helpful, therefore, for you to think carefully whether you are in the right job, especially if stress connected with work is making your irritable bowel worse. If your job makes you feel aggressive, hostile, inadequate or depressed, maybe it's time for a change. If you had a job that suited your personality and temperament you would probably do it well, and be well able to cope. So if you know that you could do your job much better if you really wanted to, but somehow you don't want to, then maybe you are in the wrong job. Most people are reluctant to make a major job change, but if a change is forced upon them (by redundancy for example) most are amazed at how much happier they are in the new job.

The days are long gone when most people stayed in the same type of job, and often with the same firm, for the whole of their working lives. Nowadays, the average person has three quite separate careers, working in at least three jobs in each career. So many people find themselves in the wrong job that, in the United States (and maybe also in the UK), three years is the average length of time for staying in any one job.

'But what else can I do?', you ask yourself. 'I'm trained to be a water engineer/secretary/dentist/filing clerk/dinner lady/accountant/car mechanic/machine operator. I don't know any other job. I'm too old/too young to do something else. I live in the wrong place. I can only work when the children are at school. I need the money this job brings in. I'd love to change, but . . .'

Whether you are considering moving to a new job, or even to a completely new career, a good way to start is to buy or borrow a copy of *What Color is Your Parachute?*, by Richard Nelson Bolles, updated each year, published by an American company called Ten Speed Press, and available in most good bookshops in Britain. There are several manuals on the market which aim to help people find their right niche in life, but this one is probably the most helpful and useful. By taking time to work through it, you will have a good idea of what your strengths and weaknesses are, what matters to you in a job, what is less important, what kind of people you like working with, what sort of job you should be looking for, how to go about getting it, whether re-training would be a good idea, and much, much more. Almost certainly,

71

by the time you have worked conscientiously through the book (which will take days rather than hours), you should have a good idea of what sort of job is right for you.

Other sources of guidance are careers advisory firms (look in Yellow Pages), or your local Education Authority careers department, or even your local secondary school careers office. Many local authorities are willing to share their knowledge and information sources with local people (not just school-leavers), and some even give access to computer programs which help you to see the direction you might go in. If you are not enjoying your job, think seriously about a change, especially if you think aspects of your job are making your IBS worse.

It is a myth that the high-powered executive suffers the highest levels of stress: blue-collar workers suffer considerably higher rates of stress than white-collar workers, largely due to the lack of control they have over their work, and the lack of interest and purpose they find in it. Stress-related illness is very closely connected with the amount of control and the status you connect with your job, so people whose jobs score badly on these two points are worse off. A job with too few challenges becomes boring, frustrating, and stressful.

A survey in *Which?* magazine in 1977 found that the most satisfied workers tended to be employed by a small firm where they had a responsible position, worked long hours, had lots to do, had some control over what they did, and felt their work was important and mattered to the firm. The survey also included a job satisfaction list, and those jobs that were high on the list were where people had higher-than-average control over how they did the job.

If you have a manual job, ask yourself:

- do I get enough variety in my job?
- does my job make good use of all my skills?
- do I get opportunities to make decisions about my work?
- do I feel valued by those above me?
- do I feel pride in the product I produce?
- can I take reasonable breaks, such as going to the toilet, when I want to?

If the answer to even one of these questions is NO, then your work is probably already a source of stress to you. It might be helpful if you could talk to someone about it, preferably someone who is in a position to make changes. Maybe your boss has never done the sort of job you do, so he is unaware of its particular stresses.

White-collar workers certainly don't escape lightly either. Many organizations expect their employees to become highly involved in the success of the company, and of their job in particular. Heavy investments of time and energy are demanded – working in the evening and at the weekend, travelling away from home on company business, going to work-related social activities, even being willing to move to a different area in the company's interest.

Whatever kind of work you do, things that can make a job stressful are:

- Too much work
- Too little work
- Time pressures
- Deadlines
- Unclear goals
- Poor prospects
- Low pay
- Bureaucracy
- Having no clear criteria of success
- Low status
- Isolation
- Having to make too many decisions
- Not being allowed to make enough decisions
- Physical fatigue
- Excessive travel
- Long hours
- The Boss's temperament
- New management style
- Customers, clients, patients who are hostile and demanding
- Feeling trapped
- Having to move house

- Redundancy, or fear of it
- Feeling your skills or attitudes are now outdated
- Divided loyalties
- Changes
- The consequences (monetary and career) of making mistakes
- Boredom
- Shift work
- Mistrust of those in power
- Career plateau
- Workplace politics
- Sexual harassment
- Bullies
- Smokers

Physical stressors at work can be:

- An unsuitable desk, chair, stool, workbench
- Working in an uncomfortable position
- Lighting that is too dim, or flickers
- Uncomfortable workwear
- Temperature too hot or too cold
- Fumes
- Eye strain
- Noise

Despite all these potential sources of stress, most people enjoy their jobs most of the time, and are happy staying there for the time being. Your irritable bowel may be one of the clearest signs you get about how you are feeling, and if your job includes too many things from these lists, perhaps you should consider a change. But don't expect any new job to be perfect; almost every job has its down-side, and before you leap from the job you know with all its imperfections, it is worth thinking carefully what it is you are trying to get away from. The job may well be extremely stressful, but your personality, beliefs and attitudes also play an important part in how you manage stress, both at work and at home.

Meal times

Here is another area where you could start to do things differently. Like so many people, IBS sufferers tend to rush around first thing in the morning, have nothing more nourishing than a cup of coffee for breakfast, followed by midday meal of those three Cs: coffee, crisps, and a cigarette. Perhaps there is more of the same during the afternoon, and finally this gastronomically delightful day ends with a large meal of all the wrong things, washed down with rather too much alcohol. Is it surprising your bowel protests!

Each new day dawns full of hope that things could be better. Make the most of it, and, starting from tomorrow's dawn, decide on some changes.

If your breakfast is always rushed, the only really logical solution (however difficult) is to get up a bit earlier. If you find getting up difficult at any time, you'll probably know that it's not much harder getting up half an hour earlier than getting up at your present time; and if you had that extra half-hour you could have a much calmer morning for very little extra effort.

So, from tomorrow morning, you will get up 30 minutes earlier than usual! Put aside all thoughts of a mere cup of coffee and a cigarette, or of a huge fry-up, and have a bowel-friendly breakfast of stewed fruit, or muesli, with some wholemeal toast, and one cup of tea or coffee (unless you know any of these disagree with you). Eat it sitting down on a proper chair at a proper table, not perched on a stool at a breakfast bar which simply encourages you to finish the meal as quickly as possible and rush on to the next thing. Take your time – after all, you've got 30 extra minutes now.

Your next stop is a visit to the toilet. When you start to eat, a 'food-now-entering-stomach' message is sent to the brain, which triggers a whole series of gastrointestinal activities as each batch of food already in the system is moved on to make room for the latest meal. All yesterday's food (and probably the food from the previous day too) that is in your large intestine gets moving, and inevitably some of it heads for the rectum, producing the familiar 'it's time for a bowel movement' feeling. This feeling is strongest in the morning, after the first meal of the day, and it an unwise man or woman who ignores these body messages.

When the waste products enter the rectum, they are surrounded by a layer of slippery mucus, which makes the stools easier to pass. If you are so busy in the morning that you won't find time for a visit to the toilet after breakfast, this mucus becomes reabsorbed back into the wall of the rectum, and the stools become hard and dry and difficult to pass. If you then wait until mid-morning or even later, don't be surprised if the simple act of having a bowel movement is not as easy as it should be. So work with your body, not against it.

All the way through the day, listen to what your body is trying to tell you. If you are tired, try to pause for a while to recoup some energy. If you are hungry, eat a nutritious meal, and stop when you feel full. Laugh when you are happy; cry when you are sad. Everything we feel is a symptom, a sign that the body is trying to tell us something. Be aware of it.

If you suspect that the food you eat is contributing in some way to your irritable bowel syndrome, try to make some changes. My book *The Irritable Bowel Diet Book* (Sheldon, 1990) has lots of recipes for different meals, all quick, easy and cheap to produce. It will also help you decide whether you need a high-fibre diet or a low-fibre diet, and how to pinpoint problem foods. Once you know what foods make your IBS worse, try hard to avoid them for a while, to give your intestines a rest, and you may find that after a few months you can eat them again without too much difficulty. You are asking for trouble if you continually abuse your insides with food they don't like.

Daily stress: the telephone

How many times a day do you rush to answer the phone, grab the handpiece, and feel your blood pressure rise as you give your name or number? Next time the phone rings – WAIT. Let it ring two or three times while you spend a moment breathing out with a long out-breath, let the in-breath come in naturally, then allow yourself another long out-breath. Be aware of any tension in your muscles, and consciously relax your face, jaw, neck, shoulders and hands. Even if you are right beside the phone, pause, and prepare yourself to answer it calmly.

If you have to make a call that is worrying you, write down in advance the points you wish to make, prepare a list of phrases that you could use, and above all relax and stay calm.

Daily stress: the car

The car is a source of much stress in our lives. Stress comes from two main sources: other drivers (how they drive, how they behave), and pressure of time (traffic jams, red lights, not being able to park, feeling rushed). Here are some ideas for managing the stress these situations can cause:

Other drivers

There's not a lot you as an individual can do to improve how others drive and behave (unless you are a driving instructor, in which case you have marvellous opportunities to teach people to drive calmly and courteously). If you get wound up by other people's driving, try to consider why this is. Why do lorry drivers make you feel so angry? Or women drivers? Or drivers of a particular make of car? Try to analyse your reactions, and see if you can become more accepting.

If you are at the receiving end of a driver's abuse or bad driving, above all *stay calm*. However tempting it might be to retaliate, just relax, accept the situation, and do the simple exercise on page 66. Next time someone shouts at you, or tries to show his superiority in some way, or feels the need to prove something at your expense, say to yourself 'This person has a problem. It is his problem. It is not my problem'. (As the Americans say, 'He has an *Additood Prarblem*'.) But that is something he must live with, and you mustn't let it bother you. You do not have that problem. Comfort yourself that, if he is a really selfish aggressive driver, one day he will get his come uppance!

Pressure of time

This all stems back to allowing enough time for the journey, hold-ups and all. However difficult it may seem, try not to be in a hurry; delays happen on the best regulated journeys, and can cause your blood pressure to increase, your tolerance to decrease, and your intestines to tie themselves in knots. For every journey, allow enough time, and then a bit more. Don't say to yourself, 'The journey takes 20 minutes, I have to be there at 2.45 pm, so I'll get ready to leave at 2.25 pm', quite forgetting that you must get your things together, get to the car, start the car, and drive off, and at the other end you must find somewhere to park, get your things out of the car, and walk into your destination – late! In an ideal world your thoughts would go something like this: 'I have to be there at 2.45 pm. It will take about five minutes to get my things together and get to the car; at the other end I must allow 5 minutes to park, collect my things, and walk to my destination. So I should leave at 2.15 pm, but in order to be quite relaxed about roadworks, amber traffic lights, and a slow lorry in front of me I'll add an extra five minutes and leave at 2.10 pm.' If, in addition, parking is likely to be a problem, add another ten minutes and leave at 2.0 pm. If you arrive too early, give yourself permission to sit in the car and relax quietly.

Managing time

It could be that your IBS is partly caused by the stress of being under pressure of time, trying to fit too many things into too short a time, at home, at work, and even at leisure. Have you thought what changes you could make to give yourself a quieter life?

'Time management' is part of today's jargon – another buzzword. It involves learning how to make the best use of your time to get everything done without it all getting on top of you. Your library or bookseller may have a book on time-management techniques. A simple approach is to list all the tasks you have to do today, or this week or this month and give them each a priority A, B or C. If you can't decide whether something should be A or B, put B. If you can't decide whether it should be B or C, put C. Then take all the As and put them in priority A1, A2, A3 . . . then all the Bs into B1, B2, B3 . . . and so on. The priorities can always be changed. Using this technique prevents you spending time on C and then feeling stressed because you haven't done A. If possible, include some relaxing pleasant activities into each category. At the end of the period, don't worry if you haven't got round to doing the Cs – if they were unimportant it doesn't matter, if they were important they will rise to become Bs.

This simple method of time management is effective whether you are the director of a multinational company or 'just a housewife'. And by using it you are beginning to control your own life, rather than let events control you.

If you often seem to have too much work for the time available, see if you can delegate some of it. Start by making a list of 'Jobs at work' or 'Jobs at home' that you would like to hand over to someone else. Think about how and when you could ask this person, and the form of words you could use. At home it might be possible to pay someone to do these jobs – housework, ironing, mowing the lawn, cleaning the car, decorating the bathroom. Or perhaps you could swop with someone ('I'll mow your lawn if you'll do my ironing'). If there are any jobs left on your list that you can neither delegate nor swop – nor pay someone to do, then perhaps doing them with someone else might make them seem less onerous; or doing them less often; or doing them all at once followed by 'rewarding' yourself.

In many cases, actually doing the job is not as bad as thinking about it. If you have to do a job you don't like, start with the easy bit of it, before going on to the worst bit. If you need to stop in the middle, try to choose a point at which it is easy (rather than difficult) to start again. But try to build difficult parts in with the easy parts, because if you do all the easiest bits first you are then left with all the awful bits, and it's tempting to go on putting them off.

Another approach to difficult jobs is to set yourself an exact time (such as 11.30 am on Thursday) and just get on and do it then. Or if it is a tangible job that you don't like (like the ironing), decide you will do it for a certain length of time – say, half an hour – and then you will stop. Whatever the task, and whatever the method you use to make yourself do it, reward yourself when it is done.

Other suggestions for organizing your time more effectively are:

- Try to do routine tasks together at the same time once a day, whether it is the ironing at home or routine paperwork at the office. By doing similar tasks in one batch they will seem to get done quicker.
- When you are doing one job, remove evidence of all the other jobs that are waiting to be done and that are simply a stressful reminder of all the work you still have to do.
- Build into your day some time for important jobs that may crop up unexpectedly, and that simply must be fitted in. If you have no time to fit them in you will soon start to feel stressed.
- Have a balanced mixture of dull and interesting jobs, of tiring and invigorating ones.
- Make time for yourself each day.
- Try to finish each job before going on to the next; but accept that not all jobs can be finished in the time allowed.
- See if some of the jobs you don't enjoy can be done by someone else who would enjoy doing them.
- When planning your day, make sure you do jobs that need a lot of energy or time or concentration when you are feeling fresh.
- If you are constantly putting off doing something, try to work out why. What exactly don't you like about that job? See if you can get help from some source. But if you really have no option but to do it, then set yourself a fixed time, and do it then. The longer you put it off, the longer it hangs over you, and it becomes a source of stress and worry.

You can probably think of many more ways in which, by doing things differently, you could feel quieter within yourself. Once you have thought about it, have the courage to put these ideas into practice. Just choose one at a time, starting with the easy ones, and when you know you can change simple things you will feel motivated to change others.

10

Building Personal Resources

To what extent, you may wonder, are your personality and your irritable bowel syndrome linked together? Could it be that the sort of person you are is affecting how your body behaves?

In her excellent book *A Woman in your own Right – Assertiveness and You*, Anne Dickson (see page 92) identifies four personality types. Although they are all women, the descriptions could fit men just as well:

Agnes is aggressive. She is loud, forceful, and seeks to enhance her own status through belittling others. She doesn't consider other people's views, and often alienates those around her. She is determined to win every situation. Agnes needs to prove her superiority by putting down other people, because underneath she is lacking in real self-esteem. Some people respond aggressively towards her, but most feel defensive; she leaves them feeling hurt, humiliated and resentful. Many people would like to get their own back on her, but are afraid to for fear of how she will treat them.

Dulcie is a doormat, who tends to opt out of all conflict. She finds it difficult to make decisions, has a persistently negative outlook on life, and sees herself as a victim of unfairness and injustice. She is great at putting herself down. Dulcie avoids taking responsibility for making choices in her life, leaving others to do that for her, which may make them frustrated and resentful.

Ivy is indirectly aggressive. She is skilled at hurting and deceiving others without their being quite able to pinpoint just how she has done it; other people, understandably, feel confused and frustrated. She doesn't trust herself or anyone else, and so will deny her real feelings. She, too, has low self-esteem, and in order to avoid rejection or hurt she needs to control and manipulate other people, and they detect her continuing undercurrent of disapproval. Her main weapon is making others feel guilty so she gets what she wants.

In all three women, their behaviour can be traced back to a lack of self-esteem. Perhaps as a child Agnes had to prove herself better than other people in order to earn love from her parents and approval from her teachers. She feels no real self-confidence in being herself, so mistrusts others. Maybe Dulcie was criticized so often as a child that she is now afraid to show her real feelings. Perhaps Ivy learned that direct straightforward behaviour is not encouraged in women, and that she must use subtle and devious ways to get what she wants.

Which one, or combination of these, are you. A bit of Agnes sometimes? Something of Dulcie? Ivy from time to time? Don't feel guilty or blame yourself for whichever you are. Just notice how you tend to behave. Your behaviour, like these three women's, almost certainly stems from how you were treated as a child. In which of these categories would you put your mother, or your father? How they behaved towards you will have programmed how you see yourself. And it is how you see yourself that determines how you behave towards other people.

Anne Dickson's fourth woman is **Selma**:

She is neither aggressive, nor over-passive, but assertive. She respects herself and other people, accepts her own positive and negative qualities, and doesn't feel the need to put others down in order to feel comfortable in herself. She can recognize her needs and ask openly and directly; if she is refused, she does not feel demolished by the rejection, because her self-esteem is secure.

All these women, and their male equivalents, will obviously feel stress from time to time, but they will handle it quite differently.

The aggressive person (who probably has an underlying insecurity and self-doubt inside that hostile exterior) will tend to expend his aggression on those around him – outbursts of temper, aggressive driving, rushing around from A to B, all the time denying that he is stressed, but that even if he is he certainly hasn't got the time to do anything about it right now. He is possibly coping quite well with his IBS, although he almost certainly denies that it is stress-related.

The passive doormat of a person (whose insecurity and lack of self-esteem is there for all to see) will turn his stress inwards into himself, because he is too afraid to risk annoying or hurting other people. He will get tense, work all the harder to prove to himself that he can do it really, inwardly blaming other people for his rotten luck while outwardly putting a brave face on it, so that people might be surprised that he was under any sort of stress. He may feel that people have taken advantage of his good nature, and be angry with himself for not having the strength of character to say NO.

Both these characters should not be surprised if they suffer from a stress-related disease, whether IBS or something else. Even though their basic personalities are determined genetically, and reinforced through childhood, adolescence and beyond, they can still learn techniques to cope with stress whether the stress is hurled outwards at other people, or pushed inwards. Both can be equally destructive.

In between is the person who is a mixture of the other two – inwardly fairly angry, but outwardly passive. He conceals his feelings, bottles up his anger, and is then surprised that he develops a stress-related condition. But IBS is very common among people who appear to be unemotional, organized and in control rather than obviously aggressive. They are often quite set in their ways, and don't like change. They turn their stress inwards like the passive person, rather than outwards like the aggressive person.

Vulnerability: passiveness and low self-esteem

Vulnerable people tend to have many of these characteristics:

- saying Yes when they want to say No
- don't like refusing other people's requests
- don't find it easy to express their feelings

- bottle things up
- feel people take advantage of them
- may be anxious and easily depressed
- worry
- sensitive and easily hurt
- tendency to erect an invisible wall around them to keep out the world's problems
- lack confidence
- a boring, unchallenging job
- difficulty in relaxing
- lacking energy
- tendency to dwell on negative things and expect the worst
- indecisiveness
- don't feel in control of their life or their health

Despite this list of apparently rather negative qualities, people like this tend to be well-liked by friends and colleagues, are easy to get along with, can be good friends to others, and are always willing to help.

So if you feel you are a passive, vulnerable person, don't have a low opinion of yourself because you are not thrusting and aggressive – your qualities are much valued. People are not judging you as harshly as you judge yourself – quite the opposite, you are almost certainly a much-valued friend and colleague.

But if . . .

Perhaps you wish you were more attractive, sophisticated, clever, bold, forceful and dynamic. Maybe you are waiting for some future time when everything will be different – when you are richer, more successful, married, have children, when the children have left home . . . in fact you find it quite hard to enjoy the here-and-now.

This is where self-talk can be so powerful, both positively and negatively. Self-talk is those things we say to ourselves:

'I'm not as attractive as her'
'Nothing ever goes right for me'
'It's all so unfair'

'I knew I should have said NO'
'I can't help how I feel'
'I must put other people's needs before my own'
'I mustn't show I'm feeling upset and angry'
'I'm like this because it runs in the family'
'How can people treat me like this?'

And so on, and on, and on. You can probably think of many more that are directly relevant to you.

But you needn't say these sorts of things to yourself. Each time your self-talk niggles away at your self-esteem, think up a positive statement that is the opposite of what you were thinking. Repeat it several times a day, and gradually you will 'accentuate the positive, eliminate the negative'. Possible examples are:

'People at work like me'
'I can make things happen the way I want them to'
'Even if something upsets me, I can make sure I do not remain upset for long'
'I can learn to change how I feel and respond to situations; I do not have to let them worry me'
'I can accept myself for what I am'
'I have the right to express how I feel'
'Everyone makes mistakes sometimes; I don't make any more mistakes than other people do'
'Lots of things about me are very attractive and likeable'
'Losers let it happen; winners make it happen'

These are just some examples of how the things you say to yourself can affect how you feel.

When your self-esteem is high, you will feel less vulnerable, and vice versa. Your self-esteem is your evaluation of yourself, and you should use all your self-talk and positive thinking to keep that evaluation high. If you place a high value on being slim, or successful in business, or good at tennis, or having successful children, and you are none of these, then your self-esteem will suffer. Try to re-order your priorities so that what you are good at is important to you; there are things about you that people like and envy, so build on them to keep your self-esteem high.

From now on give yourself permission to:

- Change your mind
- Express your feelings
- Say NO when you want to
- Be the person you are
- Distance yourself from other people's problems
- Have needs and wants
- Make mistakes
- Be the judge of your own actions
- and Do all these things without giving any reason.

Aggressiveness

Aggressive people are not good for themselves, or for those they live and work with. Aggression increases your blood pressure, your risk of coronary heart disease, your level of stress, your risk of accidents, and your chance of getting a stress-related condition. It contributes to marriage breakdown, domestic stress, alcoholism, discord at work, violence, road accidents, and much much more.

In the early 1970s, Friedman and Rosenman studied over 3400 American men who had suffered from coronary heart disease. No less than 85% of them had a personality type that the two researchers called Type A. The results of their research were published in a book called *Type A Behavior and Your Heart* which should be compulsory reading for all those who want to ensure that their aggressive personality doesn't lead them to an early grave. As many sufferers of IBS have this type of personality it could usefully have been called 'Type A Behaviour and Your Irritable Bowel'!

Type A (aggressive) people have many of these characteristics:

- hostility
- competitiveness
- quarrelsomeness
- restlessness

- impatience
- gabble talking
- swear freely
- feel under constant pressure of time
- strive for achievement
- ambition
- hard-driving
- preoccupation with deadlines
- seldom reach their goals because they continually create new ones
- inability to delegate for fear of losing control
- believe they work more effectively under pressure
- over-sensitive to criticism
- dominate the conversation
- hold stereotyped generalizations about groups
- obsessively punctual
- despise those who are slow or perform inadequately

Do many of these characteristics describe you? If so, don't ignore it. In the US, Type A behaviour is taken as a serious risk factor, about which something can and should be done. Type A people (who are very much more likely to be men than women) meet in groups to help each other. They are taught to modify their behaviour, and this improves their relationships with other people, and reduces their high risk of heart attack. Members of the group discuss how they have reacted to particular situations, and they work out how they could have reacted better, without impatience or anger, so that next time they will handle the situation better.

If you are a Type A person, there are many things about you that people like: you are self-assured, efficient, enthusiastic, and interesting, and these are qualities worth building on. But if you can be aware of those other characteristics that people may not like (being hostile, tense, quarrelsome, aggressive, impatient etc.) and try to control them, you could have the best of all worlds. Most people prefer people who are pleasant, friendly, accepting, helpful, co-operative, open, relaxed, and warm.

You too could be like this. You may feel you don't want to lose your competitive edge, or to feel so calm you don't get things done on time. You don't need to. You can simply learn to be less Type A without going too far the other way.

Like the vulnerable, passive people, you probably engage in self-talk, too, and it could be reinforcing your basic aggressive personality:

'I am very ambitious'
'I drive myself hard'
'I can't stand incompetence and inefficiency'
'I need to win to prove what I am'
'Making mistakes is a sign of weakness'
'So is admitting that you don't know something'
'Showing affection is only for wimps'
'The job will be done much better if I do it myself'
'Using strong language means I am strong'

And so on. Yet, by changing those things you say to yourself, you could become less Type A while still retaining your strengths.

'Because I am a strong person, I can afford to show affection'
'Everyone makes mistakes, and no one will think less of me if I do so too'
'Delegating a job is the sign of a responsible manager'
'I don't need to prove I am strong'
'If someone does a job slower than I do, I can accept that calmly'
'It's OK to be gentle, slow, wrong, last . . .'
'I can admit my mistakes'
'I can learn from other people'
'If I get something wrong I will not be a failure'
'Waiting is a *gift* of time, not a *waste* of time'

Give yourself permission to:

● Be wrong
● Ask for help

- Hug someone
- Do a job slowly
- Be late
- Cry
- Come second, or even last
- Remain silent
- Enjoy birds singing, water flowing, children playing
- Fail
- Feel frightened
- Let other people make decisions
- Drive slowly
- Relax

In their book, Friedman and Rosenman say, 'If you are overly hostile, certainly the most important drill measure you should adopt is that one in which you remind yourself of the fact that you are hostile'. And having done that, resolve to do things differently! Modifying your behaviour won't make you a wimp or boring, because your basic interesting personality is still there. But it may make life calmer and less stressful for your family and workmates, and it should reduce your chances of getting coronary heart disease, and also improve your IBS.

Assertiveness: the right balance

Imagine these two situations:

Your friend tells you she has had the offer of a job, but she wouldn't get home until about 6pm, and she has come to ask you if you would be able to collect her son from school every day and keep him with you until she gets home. She says there's no one else she could ask, and if you can't have her son she will have to turn down the job. You greatly value her friendship, but you really don't want to be committed to having him every day after school. If you say 'No' you risk losing a friendship that is important to you, but if you say 'Yes' you will probably resent the commitment involved, and feel annoyed with your friend for asking you, and with yourself for agreeing to do it.

You are involved in a minor road collision with another driver, and both cars receive some damage. You think it's his fault, he thinks it's yours. He is angry, aggressive and personally insulting about your driving. Do you shout back at him, giving as good as you get, his aggression matched only by yours? Or do you take his insults without retaliating, and then when you get home feel indescribably angry that he should have been so aggressive and that you let him get away with it?

Both these situations are likely to get your irritable bowel working overtime during the following few days, but there is a solution that can help you, your friend, the other driver, and your gut. It's called assertiveness.

A few years ago, a group that I belonged to decided to take a course in assertiveness training. I didn't know what it was, and I wasn't particularly interested, but as everyone else had signed on I decided to follow the crowd. It turned out to be one of the most valuable things I have ever done. Like so many people, I often wish I had been able to express myself differently on a particular occasion – perhaps more positively, perhaps less aggressively – and assertiveness training taught me how to. I don't get it right every time, but there are now fewer occasions when I feel I have said 'Yes' when I wanted to say 'No', or antagonized someone by using inappropriate words.

There have probably been many occasions when you knew you used the wrong words or the wrong tone of voice or chose the wrong time to say something; when you felt you didn't have a full opportunity to say how you felt; when you felt unable to express how you felt; when you were afraid of provoking a wrong reaction in someone else; when you expected that person to respond in one way and he or she responded quite differently. From all these situations you may retire hurt, bruised, angry or frustrated, yet not know how to make sure it doesn't happen again. In fact the more hurt and angry you are the harder it becomes to use an understanding tone of voice or considerate words.

The person who uses an aggressive manner puts his wants, needs and rights above those of other people. He tries to get his own way by not allowing others a choice. His behaviour may be active or passive, direct or indirect, honest or dishonest, but it always communicates the appearance of superiority. He wins, others lose, which can all too easily lead to a situation where others want to get their own back.

At the opposite extreme is behaviour which communicates a message of inferiority, the person who always gives in to others, the doormat, the victim. He allows the wants, needs and rights of other people to be more important than his own. Others win, he loses.

But there is a middle way – assertiveness. The assertive person communicates respect for himself and others. His wants, needs and rights are equal to other peoples'. He will influence, listen and negotiate in a way that causes others to co-operate willingly, with no desire to retaliate. With assertiveness, both sides 'win'.

As you may now see, assertiveness is not aggressiveness. It is not dominating other people, nor being dominated. It is not being unfeminine, unmasculine, overbearing, ruthless or hostile. There is a tendency for men to think they should be aggressive and women shouldn't, an assumption that often causes conflict. An assertive woman is not an aggressive woman. She may get her own way, or she may allow others to have their own way, but it will be a WIN-WIN situation, not one side winning while the other side loses.

This book is about irritable bowel syndrome and stress, and it is not possible here to teach assertiveness. But it is a skill almost everyone can benefit from. In many areas classes are held to teach the technique, often all-women or all-men groups, so that the environment is relaxed and unthreatening. Subjects that might be covered in an assertiveness course are:

- making requests
- saying NO to other people's requests and feeling all right about it
- giving criticism, and compliments
- receiving criticism, and compliments
- expressing your own anger
- handling other peoples' anger

- body language
- self-confidence and self-esteem
- resolving conflicts
- assertiveness and your children

If you are unable to find a group, two very useful books are: *When I say NO I feel guilty*, by Manuel J. Smith, published by Bantam, and *A Woman in your own Right – Assertiveness and You*, by Anne Dickson, published by Quartet Books. If you have never thought about assertiveness before, it will open up to you a whole new way of responding to other people which will benefit you for the rest of your life.

11

And Finally . . .

In a contemplative fashion, And a tranquil frame of mind,
Free from ev'ry kind of passion, Some solution let us find.
Let us grasp the situation, Solve the complicated plot –
Quiet, calm deliberation disentangles ev'ry knot.

from 'The Gondoliers', by Gilbert & Sullivan

IBS affects a significant proportion of the population. It takes up
a great deal of medical time. It causes pain, embarrassment and
worry. It remains a problem searching for a solution.

For some people the underlying cause is diet, for others it is
stress, and for some it is something unknown. Research is going
on at an encouraging rate, but still no one fully knows what it is,
what causes it, or how to cure it. One day things will change . . .
but don't hold your breath!

If you want to know more about IBS, my earlier book *Coping
Successfully with Your Irritable Bowel* (Sheldon, 1988) covers
such subjects as what it is, how you (and your doctor) can tell if
you have it, different tests and treatments, how to cope with
pain, diarrhoea, constipation and wind, stress and relaxation,
food and diet, how it may particularly affect women, the role of
alternative medicine, and much more. It also lists the guidelines
for diagnosis, so that when your doctor says 'What you've got is
irritable bowel syndrome' you will believe him and not worry
that you might have something much more serious.

For those people whose IBS may be triggered by what they
eat, *The Irritable Bowel Diet Book* (Sheldon, 1990) discusses
problem foods and how they affect IBS, food allergy and food
intolerance, different diets (high fibre, low fibre and exclusion
diets), and has lots of recipes that should make it much easier to
cook and eat for an irritable bowel.

Until very recently there was no self-help group for IBS
sufferers in the UK, but in 1991 the IBS NETWORK was

started in Sheffield. The network produces a newsletter called *Gut Reaction*, and you can find out more about it from:

Susan Backhouse
IBS Network
c/o Voluntary Action Sheffield
General Office
69 Division Street
SHEFFIELD S1 4GE

If you want to know where your nearest IBS self-help group is, or if you are interested in starting one in your area, write to:

Christine Dancey
c/o The Wells Park Health Project
1a Wells Park Road
Sydenham
LONDON SE26 6JE

If you write to either of these addresses, please enclose an s.a.e. for a reply.

The first issue of the IBS Newsletter *Gut Reaction* was produced early in 1991. The editorial said:

As a newsletter produced by and for sufferers of Irritable Bowel Syndrome, it is a first in this country. It is an important step in the right direction for improving things for people with this disorder. Many sufferers do not meet with much understanding from doctors, friends and family. Although it is gradually being taken more seriously by those in the medical profession there is a long way to go, and they still know very little about the condition.

We hope this newsletter will provide sufferers with a chance to read about other people's experiences, to learn about ways of helping themselves and to improve the information available on the subject.

Many people don't know anyone else who suffers from IBS and can feel alone, embarrassed, depressed and worried about what may be wrong with them. It is possible that these feelings may make the symptoms worse.

We feel more needs to be done to help people understand the disorder. Sufferers need to be given information so they can help themselves, and more research needs to be done into the causes and possible 'cures'.

You are not alone. There are thousands like you with similar symptoms and similar anxieties. Even if conventional medicine has no cure yet, there is still a great deal you can do to help yourself, and to reduce the effect IBS has on you. If you can follow some of the ideas from this book, and be willing to make some changes, every aspect of your life will benefit.

Grant me the serenity to accept the things I cannot change,
The courage to change the things I can,
And the wisdom to know the difference.

Reinhold Niebuhr

Index

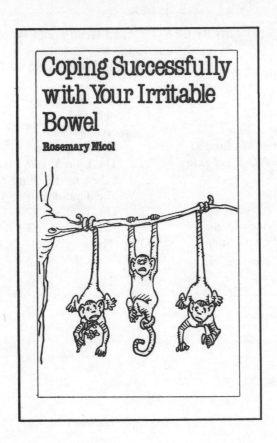

Coping Successfully with Your Irritable Bowel

Rosemary Nicol

'written sympathetically . . . the book will be a boon for all those who suffer pain and embarrassment' Virginia Ironside in *The Sunday Mirror*

'sensitively written, makes practical suggestions for dealing with abdominal pain, constipation, diarrhoea and stress, and reviews conventional and alternative treatments' *Cosmopolitan*

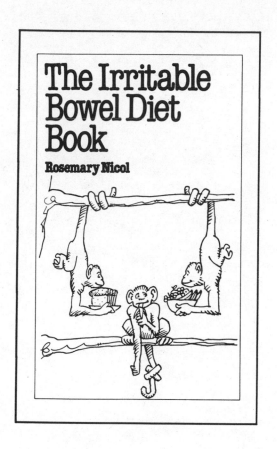

The Irritable
Bowel Diet
Book

Rosemary Nicol

A diet book that will help you cope with IBS without disrupting your life. It's packed with recipes and suggestions for healthy and enjoyable meals, and advice about what to choose for a snack lunch at work, what to order in a restaurant and how to cope when you're invited out for a meal.

Available from all good bookshops, or direct from
Sheldon Press Mail Order
36 Steep Hill, Lincoln LN2 1LU